Common Pitfalls in Cognitive and Behavioral Neurology

Common Pitfalls in Cognitive and Behavioral Neurology

A Case-Based Approach

Keith Josephs
Mayo Clinic

Federico Rodríguez-Porcel
Medical University of South Carolina

Rhonna Shatz
University of Cincinnati

Daniel Weintraub
University of Pennsylvania

Alberto Espay
University of Cincinnati

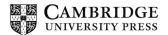
CAMBRIDGE
UNIVERSITY PRESS

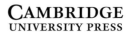

CAMBRIDGE
UNIVERSITY PRESS

University Printing House, Cambridge CB2 8BS, United Kingdom

One Liberty Plaza, 20th Floor, New York, NY 10006, USA

477 Williamstown Road, Port Melbourne, VIC 3207, Australia

314–321, 3rd Floor, Plot 3, Splendor Forum, Jasola District Centre, New Delhi – 110025, India

79 Anson Road, #06–04/06, Singapore 079906

Cambridge University Press is part of the University of Cambridge.

It furthers the University's mission by disseminating knowledge in the pursuit of education, learning, and research at the highest international levels of excellence.

www.cambridge.org
Information on this title: www.cambridge.org/9781108814157
DOI: 10.1017/9781108355841

First published 2021

Printed in the United Kingdom by TJ Books Limited, Padstow Cornwall

A catalogue record for this publication is available from the British Library.

Library of Congress Cataloging-in-Publication Data
Names: Josephs, Keith, author. | Rodriguez-Porcel, Federico, author. | Shatz, Rhonna, author. | Weintraub, Daniel, author. | Espay, Alberto J., author.
Title: Common pitfalls in cognitive and behavioral neurology : a case-based approach / Keith Josephs, Federico Rodriguez-Porcel, Rhonna Shatz, Daniel Weintraub, Alberto Espay.
Description: Cambridge, United Kingdom ; New York, NY : Cambridge University Press, 2020. | Includes bibliographical references and index.
Identifiers: LCCN 2020012178 (print) | LCCN 2020012179 (ebook) | ISBN 9781108814157 paperback | ISBN 9781108355841 OC | ISBN 9781108431132 DO PB
Subjects: MESH: Neurocognitive Disorders – diagnosis | Neurobehavioral Manifestations | Neurologic Examination | Case Reports
Classification: LCC RC337 (print) | LCC RC337 (ebook) | NLM WM 40 | DDC 616.8/046072–dc23
LC record available at https://lccn.loc.gov/2020012178
LC ebook record available at https://lccn.loc.gov/2020012179

ISBN 978-1-108-81415-7 Paperback
ISBN 978-1-108-35584-1 Cambridge Core
ISBN 978-1-108-43113-2 Print/Online Bundle

To my children, Kayley, Kennedy and Kzeph. – KAJ

To my parents, Graciela and Carlos, my children, Lucas, Beatriz and Elena, and my wife, Lilie. They know why. – FRP

To my husband MWS who gives me the weekdays at UC, to my daughter AES who will write the next generation of this book, and my son BDR who should write his own book. -RS

To my wife, Suzanne, and my daughters, Sophia and Phoebe, who are my primary inspiration in life. - DW

To Carrie Roark and Lori Selm, my medical and academic assistants, for their infinite patience and support. -AJE

Contents

The colour plate section can be found between pp. 98 and 99.

Diseases Discussed in the Book

Warning: Browsing through this list with a goal other than the anticipatory reward release of dopamine may spoil the stimulating experience of navigating the cases without knowing their destination.

Disease	Cases
Alzheimer disease – amnestic variant	1, 3, 11, 29
Alzheimer disease – corticobasal syndrome	40
Alzheimer disease – frontal variant	16
Alzheimer disease – management issues	47, 48, 49, 51
Alzheimer disease – monogenic	37
Alzheimer disease – posterior cortical atrophy	10, 25
Behavioral variant of frontotemporal dementia	4, 5, 9
Behavioral variant of frontotemporal dementia – monogenic	7, 15, 27
Cerebellar cognitive/affective syndrome	22
Cerebral amyloid angiopathy-related inflammation	45
Cerebral autosomal dominant arteriopathy with subcortical infarcts and leukoencephalopathy (CADASIL)	41
Chronic traumatic encephalopathy	24
Creutzfeldt–Jakob disease	34
Dementia with Lewy bodies	8, 20, 31, 33
Fragile X associated tremor/ataxia syndrome	43
Limbic encephalitis	17
Logopenic variant of primary progressive aphasia	28
Medication-induced cognitive impairment	38
Multifactorial cognitive impairment	35
Multiple sclerosis	30
Multiple system atrophy	23
Niemann Pick type C	18
Normal pressure hydrocephalus	42
Occipital epilepsy	26
Parkinson disease – depression	2
Parkinson disease – fluctuations	19, 39
Parkinson disease – hydrocephalus	50
Parkinson disease – impulse control disorder	46
Post-HSV anti-NMDA-R encephalitis	32
Primary progressive apraxia of speech	21
Semantic variant of primary progressive aphasia	6, 14
Sleep apnea–induced cognitive impairment	36
Subdural hematoma	13
Suspected non–Alzheimer disease pathophysiology (SNAP)	44
Transient epileptic amnesia	12

Preface

Understanding how humans perceive, interpret, and interact with the world has attracted some of the most brilliant minds in history. The existence of this book is an indication that it still does. While sophisticated diagnostic and experimental methods to better understand the nervous system in health and disease continue to flourish, all of the exciting knowledge and hypotheses have the same origin and destination: the patient.

Keen observation and insightful questions have been sparked from single cases. Recognition of the role of the mesial temporal lobe in memory encoding came from learning about patient "H.M."; of the prefrontal cortex in behavior, from Phineas Gage; of the left inferior frontal cortex in language, from patient "Tan." Scientific endeavors without a connection with patients' challenges may never help in understanding those challenges, much less alleviating them.

For clinicians, no knowledge of a disease is more poignant than when it comes from a patient experience, particularly if errors in observation or interpretation of data led to incorrect diagnostic or therapeutic decisions. Because the practice of neurology is fraught with potential pitfalls, this book became an opportunity to catalog them into examination oversights, diagnostic misinterpretation, and therapeutic misadventures. Through the wisdom of hindsight, the reader will appreciate many case-based educational sessions uncovering diagnoses missed or wrongly attributed, cognitive disorders difficult to characterize, tests inappropriately ordered or interpreted, and treatments incorrectly chosen or dosed. As with the other books in the Common Pitfalls series, the lessons generated from these highly selected cases can become powerful and enduring, informing and enhancing clinical practice.

In selecting the cases for each of the chapters, we took care in emphasizing those with lessons beyond the specific pitfalls exposed, highlighting gaps in knowledge and even areas of controversy. While there was an inherent bias toward neurodegenerative disorders, given the scope of our practice, we have made every effort to include other neurological disorders. Each of the authors took turns at feeling uneasy on matters related to interpretation of data from the literature on a given case, and attempted to lay bare the area of weakness. We admittedly "sanitized" many cases of the messy data from which they emerged, writing each with only the relevant details, in a sequence that succinctly brought order to the corresponding pitfall. Of course, clinical decision making for our patients may not look like that enacted in the chapters if only to maximize concentration on the aspects that hide the pearls of wisdom.

That each of the five authors came from different but complementary backgrounds was deliberately meant to reflect the breadth of cognitive and behavioral neurology practice and to ensure all angles were appropriately covered. As a result, we each also learned from one another in writing this book. We hope that the challenges we faced and the knowledge we gained as we worked on the *Common Pitfalls* compendium will equally translate into the reader's experience.

Although we tried to minimize it, some dose of redundancy was unavoidable when considering all pitfalls, given the inherent overlap between some. When the same or a related disorder is brought up in different chapters, we refer the reader to these complementary sections to enhance the educational value. For instance, difficulties in the recognition of certain frontotemporal dementias may come from neglecting helpful clinical signs or from missing neuroimaging clues, pitfalls addressed in different chapters. Notwithstanding any overzealous cross-referencing, this book is meant to be read in any order and at any pace. According to the Common Pitfalls style, each individual case stands on its own.

This book is published at a time when the foundations of cognitive and behavioral neurology are being challenged. Biomarker development is slowly moving from disease constructs (convergence biomarkers; applicable to most) to individuals with those diseases (divergence biomarkers; present in some but absent in most of those with the same clinical disease). The separation between neurodegenerative disorders long made across clinico-pathologic boundaries is slowly reorganizing across genetic–molecular domains. Consequently, much of what we conceive today in terms of nosology may be different in the future. Until then, this book will remain a testament to the value of curiosity and critical thinking applied to the care of individual patients with cognitive or behavioral disorders.

Keith Josephs

Federico Rodríguez-Porcel

Rhonna Shatz

Daniel Weintraub

Alberto Espay

Acknowledgements

The authors thank first and foremost our patients for their challenges is the source and goal of this book. In addition, we thank Drs. Jose Biller, Marcelo Kauffman, Jorge Ortiz-Garcia, David Riley and Sergio Rodriguez-Quiroga for providing some illustrative cases discussed in this book. We are also grateful to Nick Dunton, Senior Commissioning Editor at Cambridge University Press, who encouraged us to take this challenge and the other colleagues at Cambridge, Katy Nardoni, Camille Lee-Own, Gayathri Tamilselvan, for their editorial support.

Abbreviations

ACB	anticholinergic burden	CSF	cerebrospinal fluid
AD	Alzheimer disease	CTE	chronic traumatic encephalopathy
ADC	apparent diffusion coefficient	DAWS	dopamine agonist withdrawal syndrome
ADLs	activities of daily living		
AE	autoimmune encephalitis	DDS	dopamine dysregulation syndrome
AHI	apnea/hypopnea index	DESH	disproportionately enlarged subarachnoid space hydrocephalus
ALS	amyotrophic lateral sclerosis		
AOS	apraxia of speech	DLB	dementia with Lewy bodies
APOE	apolipoprotein E	DLBD	diffuse Lewy body disease
ATI	amyloid β-42/total tau index	DWI	diffusion-weighted image
ATL	anterior temporal pole	EBV	Epstein–Barr virus
AVLT	auditory verbal learning test	ECT	electroconvulsive therapy
BDI	Beck Depression Inventory	EM	episodic memory
BP	blood pressure	EOAD	early-onset Alzheimer disease
bvFTD	behavioral variant of frontotemporal dementia	FBDS	faciobrachial dystonic seizures
		FBI	Frontal Behavioral Inventory
CAA	cerebral amyloid angiopathy	FDBS	faciobrachial dystonic seizures
CADASIL	cerebral autosomal dominant arteriopathy with subcortical infarcts and leukoencephalopathy	FDG-PET	fluorodeoxyglucose positron emission tomography
		FrSBe	Frontal Systems Behavioral Scale
CAF	Clinician Assessment of Fluctuation	FTLD	frontotemporal lobar degeneration
CASPR2	contactin-associated protein 2	FUS	fused in sarcoma
CBD	corticobasal degeneration	fvAD	frontal variant of Alzheimer disease
CBS	corticobasal syndrome		
CBS-AD	corticobasal syndrome due to Alzheimer disease	FXTAS	fragile X–associated tremor-ataxia syndrome
CBS-Tau	corticobasal syndrome due to tauopathy	GDS-15	15-item version of the Geriatric Depression Scale
CBT	cognitive behavioral therapy	GRE	gradient-echo weighted
CCAS	cerebellar cognitive affective syndrome	HCA	healthy cognitive aging
		HD	Huntington disease
CDR	Clinical Dementia Rating Scale	HDRS	Hamilton Depression Rating Scale
CERAD	Consortium to Establish a Registry for Alzheimer's Disease	HES	herpes simplex encephalitis
		HIV	human immunodeficiency virus
ChEI	cholinesterase inhibitors	IADLs	instrumental activities of daily living
CJD	Creutzfeldt–Jakob disease		
CNS-LS	Center for Neurological-Study Lability Scale	ICB	impulsive-compulsive behavior
		ICD	impulse control disorder
CPAP	continuous positive airway pressure	IEM	inborn errors of metabolism

IQCODE	Informant Questionnaire on Cognitive Decline in the Elderly		PLACS	Pathological Laughing and Crying Scale
IVIG	intravenous immunoglobulin		PNH	peripheral nerve hyperexcitability
LATE	limbic associated TDP-43 encephalopathy		PPAOS	primary progressive apraxia of speech
LB	Lewy bodies		PSP	progressive supranuclear palsy
LE	limbic encephalitis		PSP-RS	Richardson syndrome variant of progressive supranuclear palsy
LGI1	glioma inactivated-1		PSWC	periodic sharp wave complexes
lvPPA	logopenic variant of primary progressive aphasia		QUIP	Questionnaire for Impulsive-Compulsive Disorders in Parkinson Disease
MBI	mild behavioral impairment		QUIP-RS	Questionnaire for Impulsive-Compulsive Disorders in Parkinson Disease Rating Scale
MBI-C	MBI checklist			
MCI	mild cognitive impairment			
MCP	middle cerebellar peduncle		RPD	rapidly progressive dementia
MMSE	Mini-Mental State Examination		RT-QuIC	real-time quaking-induced conversion
MoCA	Montreal Cognitive Assessment			
MS	multiple sclerosis		SD	semantic dementia
MSA	multiple system atrophy		SDH	subdural hematoma
MSA-C	multiple system atrophy, cerebellar type		SH	supine hypertension
			SIADH	inappropriate antidiuretic hormone secretion
MSA-P	multiple system atrophy, parkinsonian type		SM	semantic memory
MTL	medial temporal lobe		SNAP	suspected non–Alzheimer disease pathophysiology
nfvPPA	nonfluent/agrammatic variant of primary progressive aphasia		SNRI	serotonin–norepinephrine reuptake inhibitor
NMDA-R	N-methyl-D-aspartate receptor			
NMF	nonmotor fluctuations		SSRI	selective serotonin reuptake inhibitor
NPC	Niemann–Pick type C		SVD	small-vessel disease
NPH	normal pressure hydrocephalus		svPPA	semantic variant of primary progressive aphasia
NPI	Neuropsychiatric Inventory			
NPI-Q	Neuropsychiatric Inventory Questionnaire		SWI	susceptibility weighted imaging
			TDP-43	transactive response DNA binding protein 43
NPS	neuropsychiatric symptoms			
OH	orthostatic hypotension		TEA	transient epileptic amnesia
PBA	pseudobulbar affect		TGA	transient global amnesia
PCA	posterior cortical atrophy		UTI	urinary tract infection
PD	Parkinson disease		VGKCC-ab	voltage-gated potassium channel complex antibodies
PDD	Parkinson disease dementia			
PD-MCI	Parkinson disease–associated mild cognitive impairment		VH	visual hallucination
			VPS	Ventriculoperitoneal shunt
PET	positron emission tomography		YOD	young-onset dementia
PFC	prefrontal cortex			

1   It's Just Old Age

Case: This 68-year-old right-handed man was evaluated after an episode of delirium. Three months prior, in the span of two days, he became confused and agitated. At the hospital, he was found to have a urinary tract infection (UTI). Within three days after treatment, he returned to his baseline cognitive function and remained stable since. Although he initially reported no cognitive problems, upon further questioning, he acknowledged word-finding difficulties and forgetfulness for at least the previous two years. His daughter reported that he repeated questions and stories. In addition, she had been supervising his finances for the past year after he failed to pay some bills. Furthermore, he now needed to be reminded of appointments. Otherwise, he continued to function independently in terms of his other instrumental activities of daily living (IADLs) with no meaningful change since retirement as an accountant four years ago. He became a widower five years prior and was living by himself. The patient felt that most friends his age had similar issues. He and his daughter had also been reassured by their primary care physician that these issues were part of normal aging.

Given His Return to Baseline and Independent Functioning, Ostensibly Similarly to His Peers, Is It Necessary to Consider Further Investigations?

Despite his ability to lead an almost independent life, there were some concerning elements in the history. First, the episode of delirium in the context of a UTI suggested that a decrease in his cognitive reserve made him vulnerable to encephalopathy. Second, there were already "minor," but increasing, cognitive difficulties. These should be evaluated and addressed even if he was otherwise functioning well.

His general neurologic exam was unremarkable. The Montreal Cognitive Assessment (MoCA) score was 25/30 due to impairments in sentence repetition, phonemic fluency, and delayed recall (he was able to recall two out of five words freely and recognized one

additional word when multiple choices were given). A brain MRI showed cortical atrophy predominantly in the medial temporal lobe bilaterally (Figure 1.1). CSF biomarkers showed low beta-amyloid and elevated total/phosphorylated tau, suggestive of Alzheimer disease (AD).

Discussion

Healthy cognitive aging (HCA) may be associated with a decline in cognitive function. However, study of what can be considered HCA is evolving, and the understanding of the domains and extent to which they are affected remains uncertain (Table 1.1).

Although most changes seen in HCA begin around the seventh decade, a progressive decline in processing speed may begin as early as the third decade of life in healthy individuals (Salthouse, 2010). Simple attention remains stable, whereas divided attention may decline over time (Treitz et al., 2007). This may be described by individuals with HCA as having difficulties with multitasking or following multiple conversations simultaneously. Language overall remains stable through life (Park and Reuter-Lorenz, 2009). Some domains, like vocabulary, even improve with aging (Harada et al., 2013). Decline in certain types of verbal fluency may reflect changes in processing speed and retrieval deficits rather than a language impairment (Harada et al., 2013).

Overall, memory processes dependent on frontal-executive networks (e.g., working memory) may be affected in HCA, while those dependent on temporal networks are not. Overlearned knowledge, including autobiographical, semantic, and procedural memory, remain intact in HCA, while other domains experience different degrees of changes with age (Harada et al., 2013). Learning and acquisition of new memories may be affected in HCA partly due to difficulties in divided attention or filtering irrelevant information (Stevens et al., 2008). Free recall may decline in HCA, but recognition memory (i.e., with cueing) remains normal (Harada et al., 2013). Visuospatial perception (e.g., estimation of distance) is preserved with HCA, although a decline in visuospatial constructive

Table 1.1 Domains that may decline with healthy cognitive aging versus those that do not

Domain	May decline with HCA[a]	Does not decline with HCA
Attention	Divided attention	Simple attention
Executive functions	Processing speed Working memory	Set-shifting Inhibition
Language	Verbal fluency	Vocabulary Naming Repetition
Memory	Learning of new information Source memory (i.e., knowing when or where something was learned)	Recall of learned information Recognition Semantic memory Procedural memory
Visuospatial	Constructive visuospatial skills	Perceptive visuospatial skills

[a] As noted in the discussion, there is little certainty of what changes may be expected in healthy cognitive aging.

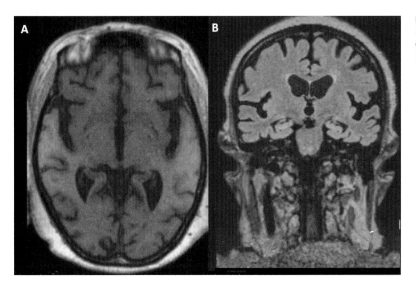

Figure 1.1 T1-weighted axial and coronal brain MRI in this patient. Note the (A) cortical atrophy and (B) medial temporal lobe atrophy.

abilities (e.g., copying a three-dimensional figure) may be observed later in life (Howieson et al., 1993).

Despite multiple studies examining HCA, the findings have been questioned, as they included patients who later developed neurodegenerative diseases (i.e., people who may have been manifesting the initial signs and symptoms of the disease process, as opposed to only those truly with healthy aging). More importantly, while group-level data help in understanding the processes underpinning aging, it is not always easy to extrapolate to individuals. Therefore any decline in cognitive function should be evaluated as a potential first sign of neurodegenerative pathology.

Diagnosis: Amnestic-type mild cognitive impairment with Alzheimer disease pathology

Tip: Healthy cognitive aging may affect certain domains (e.g., speed processing) but should never significantly affect performance in daily activities. Given the uncertain boundaries of normal and pathologic cognitive decline, a comprehensive evaluation of these individuals is warranted.

References

Harada, C. N., Natelson Love, M. C. and Triebel, K. L. 2013. Normal cognitive aging. *Clin Geriatr Med* **29**(4) 737–752.

Howieson, D. B. et al. 1993. Neurologic function in the optimally healthy oldest old: neuropsychological evaluation. *Neurology* **43**(10) 1882–1886.

Park, D. C. and Reuter-Lorenz, P. 2009. The adaptive brain: aging and neurocognitive scaffolding. *Annu Rev Psychol* **60** 173–196.

Salthouse, T. A. 2010. Selective review of cognitive aging. *J Int Neuropsychol Soc* **16**(5) 754–760.

Stevens, W. D., Hasher, L., Chiew, K. S. and Grady, C. L. 2008. A neural mechanism underlying memory failure in older adults. *J Neurosci* **28**(48) 12820–12824.

Treitz, F. H., Heyder, K. and Daum, I. 2007. Differential course of executive control changes during normal aging. *Neuropsychol Dev Cogn B Aging Neuropsychol Cogn* **14**(4) 370–393.

Case: This 65-year-old left-handed woman with a 4-year history of Parkinson disease (PD) presented with worsening ability to focus and slowness of thinking. She had initially noticed a left-hand resting tremor and slowness. Benefit from levodopa was excellent, with complete disappearance of her motor symptoms. Within the last two years, she complained of impairments in attention and multitasking. She also noticed that it took her longer to process information. She had difficulty remembering names, which she could recall after a minute or two. Her family noticed that she seemed more withdrawn and irritable. Increases of levodopa dosage were limited by development of dyskinesia, failing to provide benefit to her mobility or her cognition. On exam, she exhibited masked facies and minimal asymmetric bradykinesia. Her gait was slow with decreased arm swing and stooped posture.

On her initial evaluation three years prior, she had denied concerns regarding her cognition, validated by a Montreal Cognitive Assessment (MoCA) of 29/30 (she could not recall one word freely but could after cueing). The repeat MoCA (version 2) on this visit was 22/30 due to impairments in trail making, cube copying, phonemic fluency (she said five words within the first 10 seconds and then stopped), and delayed recall (she recalled two words freely and recognized the other three when multiple choices were given).

Given all of this information, she had been diagnosed with Parkinson disease–associated mild cognitive impairment (PD-MCI).

Can We Attribute Her Cognitive Decline to the Progression of PD?

Cognitive impairment is a common feature seen in the progression of PD. However, PD may lead to cognitive impairment through multiple mechanisms, beyond the neurodegenerative changes in cognitive networks. These include changes in mood (e.g., depression), sleep (e.g., sleep fragmentation), and autonomic function (e.g., orthostatic hypotension). Given their potential for treatment, these need to be evaluated.

She denied sadness or depression. She acknowledged that she was not sleeping well and felt fatigued during the day. Her husband did not report snoring or dream enactment behaviors. There was no postural lightheadedness, and orthostatic blood pressure measurements were negative. She was only on carbidopa/levodopa and denied the intake of alcohol or any over-the-counter sleep aids.

Can Sleep Be a Contributor? Should It Be Targeted?

Sleep deprivation can affect cognition through multiple mechanisms. However, many sleeping aids have a sedative burden, which itself may affect cognition and level of energy. Despite increasing sleep quantity, sedatives do not improve quality of sleep. It is always important to ask specifically about the use of over-the-counter sleep aids since most contain diphenhydramine, a potent anticholinergic associated with cognitive impairment.

Her story suggests neither REM sleep behavior disorder nor sleep apnea as an etiology. Depression is often unrecognized as a source of fragmented sleep architecture and should be strongly considered in this case. While the unstructured interview may miss the presence of depression, the routine use of screening questionnaires can be helpful.

The 15-item version of the Geriatric Depression Scale (GDS-15) was administered. She scored 10 points (cutoff 5), supporting the presence of depression.

Discussion

Depression is a common comorbidity in neurodegenerative diseases. In PD, up to 35 percent of patients have significant depressive symptoms (Reijnders et al., 2008). Depression may precede the onset of motor symptoms and is associated with a more rapid progression, in addition to worse quality of life and functional ability (Duncan et al., 2014; Weintraub et al., 2004). Depressed PD patients are more likely to have cognitive impairment than those without (Aarsland et al., 2010; Monastero et al., 2013). However, the cause–effect relationship between depression and cognitive impairment remains unsettled (Aarsland et al., 2014).

Depression is only identified in half of PD patients (Shulman et al., 2002). It may be challenging to identify depression in these cases because PD and depression share the same decreased attention, slowness of thought process and movement, fatigue, stooped posture, and

Table 2.1 Clinical features differentiating cognitive impairment in depression and neurodegenerative dementia

	Mood-based cognitive impairment	Neurodegenerative dementia
Onset	Variable	Insidious
Insight to deficits	Present	May be absent
Attention	Easily distractible	Preserved
Language	Preserved	Impaired
Memory	Impaired retrieval Benefits from cueing	Impaired learning, encoding, and retrieval, depending on the condition Does not benefit from cueing
Visuospatial abilities	Impairment in complex tasks	Impaired in simple and complex tasks
Praxis	Preserved	Impaired
Effort	Poor	Good
Benefit from encouragement	Significant	Poor

lack of facial expression (Timmer et al., 2017). Depression is usually underreported in PD, with only 1 percent of patients volunteering depressive symptoms (Global Parkinson's Disease Survey, 2002). Also, the presence of cognitive impairment or apathy may decrease the patient's awareness of depressive symptoms. Apathy and depression frequently coexist (Aarsland et al., 2014).

Neuropsychological testing can be very helpful in differentiating between mood-based cognitive impairment and neurodegenerative dementia (Table 2.1). In both, deficits in attention, concentration, and processing speed are proportional to the severity of the disease (Potter and Steffens, 2007). However, the structure and content of speech, temporal orientation, and basic constructive abilities remain relatively intact in depression, while they tend to deteriorate with primary neurodegeneration (Schulz and Arora, 2015). Learning and memory encoding are not affected in mood-based cognitive impairment, so the performance improves when cueing is provided, different to what is observed in neurodegenerative dementias.

Special consideration needs to be taken to avoid overlooking depression for neuropsychiatric slowness in PD or confusing it with apathy. This has led to the proposal of discarding anhedonia as a core feature of depression in neurodegenerative diseases (Aarsland et al., 2014). Moreover, the assessment of depression warrants the input from an informant as well as a screening questionnaire (e.g., Hamilton Depression Rating Scale [HDRS], Beck Depression Inventory [BDI], or Geriatric Depression Scale [GDS-15]). Fluctuation of symptoms in relationship with dopaminergic therapy needs to be assessed, as depression may represent a nonmotor fluctuation and be amenable to improvement with changes in dopaminergic stimulation.

Depression often contributes to cognitive impairment as well. Treatment of depressive symptoms may have a positive effect on cognitive function. However, when considering an antidepressant, avoiding those with anticholinergic and sedative burden is recommended (see Case 38).

Our patient was started on sertraline 50 mg, gradually increased to 150 mg. She returned after four months describing significant improvements in her mood as well as in her ability to concentrate and her processing speed. Her sleep quality also improved, so she declined a sleep study.

Diagnosis: Depression presenting as (or contributing to) cognitive impairment in Parkinson disease

Tip: Depression must always be screened for in patients with cognitive impairment, with the help of a caregiver and screening questionnaires. Empirical treatment, avoiding medications with sedative or anticholinergic burden, may be attempted.

References

Aarsland, D. et al. 2010. Mild cognitive impairment in Parkinson disease: a multicenter pooled analysis. *Neurology* **75**(12) 1062–1069.

Aarsland, D., Taylor, J. P. and Weintraub, D. 2014. Psychiatric issues in cognitive impairment. *Mov Disord* **29** (5) 651–662.

Duncan, G. W. et al. 2014. Health-related quality of life in early Parkinson's disease: the impact of nonmotor symptoms. *Mov Disord* **29**(2) 195–202.

Global Parkinson's Disease Survey Steering Committee. 2002. Factors Impacting on Quality of Life in Parkinson's Disease: Results From an International Survey. Mov Disord 17(1) 60–67.

Monastero, R. et al. 2013. The neuropsychiatric profile of Parkinson's disease subjects with and without mild cognitive impairment. *J Neural Transm (Vienna)* **120**(4) 607–611.

Potter, G. G. and Steffens, D. C. 2007. Contribution of depression to cognitive impairment and dementia in older adults. *Neurologist* **13**(3) 105–117.

Reijnders, J. S. et al. 2008. A systematic review of prevalence studies of depression in Parkinson's disease. *Mov Disord* **23** (2) 183–189; quiz 313.

Schulz, P. E. and Arora, G. 2015. Depression. *Continuum* **21** (3) 756–771.

Shulman, L. M., Taback, R. L., Rabinstein, A. A. and Weiner, W. J. 2002. Non-recognition of depression and other non-motor symptoms in Parkinson's disease. *Parkinsonism Relat Disord* **8**(3) 193–197.

Timmer, M. H. M., van Beek, M., Bloem, B. R. and Esselink, R. A. J. 2017. What a neurologist should know about depression in Parkinson's disease. *Pract Neurol* **17**(5) 359–368.

Weintraub, D. et al. 2004. Effect of psychiatric and other nonmotor symptoms on disability in Parkinson's disease. *J Am Geriatr Soc* **52**(5) 784–788.

Case: This 86-year-old right-handed man presented with a 5-year history of worsening difficulties with verbal comprehension. His family had first noticed he was less interactive in social situations. He had difficulties following conversations in larger groups, though he could still maintain conversation when talking one-on-one. Around the same time, his daughter who lived in another state, reported his increasing difficulties understanding her when they were on the phone. She tried increasing the volume of her voice to no avail. His wife needed to continuously repeat things because he did not seem to understand. At home, he would watch TV at a higher volume than usual. In addition, when he was focused on something, he seemed oblivious to what others said. He had difficulties locating sounds. Interestingly, the family noted he did not have any problems hearing the phone ring or the dog bark. His speech, language, and voice volume remained unchanged. Due to these issues, he had a hearing evaluation, which concluded he had mild presbycusis. Hearing aids were placed without significant improvement despite multiple adjustments. His family noticed he increasingly needed to be told things more than once but attributed it to his hearing impairment. When the patient was asked, he acknowledged some difficulties understanding people, particularly if there was background noise. Otherwise, he denied any other issues with memory or thinking.

On exam he exhibited moderate hearing deficit to finger rub. He was able to follow commands, though repetition of the task instructions was required occasionally.

The Montreal Cognitive Assessment (MoCA) score was 21/30 due to impairments in trail making, cube copy, sentence repetition, and delayed recall (he recalled three words freely and recognized the other two when multiple choices were given).

Can His Changes Be Attributed to a Peripheral Auditory Impairment?

Although the symptoms described have hearing as common factor, they do not automatically indicate a peripheral etiology. First, the rather preserved ability to detect simple sounds (e.g., dog barking, telephone ringing) relative to the substantial impairment in understanding more complex sounds (e.g., conversations) suggests his sound perception was not as affected as his ability to process those sounds into meaningful messages. Moreover, the use of hearing aids did not provide meaningful benefits. Finally, some of the points he missed on the MoCA, namely, cube drawing and delayed recall after intact repetition, are unlikely to be attributed to impaired hearing but rather may indicate cognitive impairment.

Further evaluation included a brain structural MRI, which showed generalized atrophy, with greater involvement of the mesial temporal lobes. Cerebrospinal fluid biomarker testing showed low aβ42 and elevated phosphorylated and total tau, supportive of the diagnosis of early Alzheimer disease.

Discussion

When presented with progressive changes in auditory function, it is important to differentiate between hearing loss (i.e., impaired detection of sound) and auditory cognition (i.e., impaired understanding of, or behavioral responses to, sound), although they may coexist (Hardy et al., 2016). While the latter is indicative of a neurodegenerative process, the former impacts cognitive performance regardless of the presence of dementia (Lin et al., 2011). Sensorineural hearing loss leads to cortical reorganization and increases cognitive load, diverting cognitive resources to auditory processing at the expense of other cognitive processes (Campbell and Sharma, 2013). As a result patients may exhibit deficits in cognitive domains, including language, working memory, and free recall (Jayakody et al., 2018; Wingfield et al., 2006). In addition, individuals with hearing impairment are at higher risk of cognitive impairment (Deal et al., 2017). Therefore, hearing loss should be considered a treatable risk factor for dementia. Auditory function must be evaluated and treated, even in the context of a clear neurodegenerative disorder.

During the clinical interview, certain features may help weigh the relative impact of peripheral and central causes of hearing impairment, although most features may be caused by either process (Table 3.1). In the latter, the ability to process more complex sounds, like speech, becomes disproportionately

Table 3.1 Clinical features helpful in discerning cognitive from isolated hearing impairment

Suggestive of isolated hearing impairment	Suggestive of cognitive impairment	May be present in both
• Lack of reaction to simple sounds • Tendency to increase the TV volume or to ask people to speak louder • Sounds becomes rapidly louder with increasing sound level (loudness recruitment)	• Disproportionate deficits in comprehending speech compared to simple sounds • Impaired ability to recognize familiar voices or sounds • Impaired prosody comprehension	• Difficulty following a conversation with background noise • Inability to locate sounds • Hallucinations and tinnitus

impaired when compared to the comprehension of simple sounds. Beyond pure word comprehension, other aspects of speech may become affected, such as the ability to understand prosody or identify familiar voices. Difficulties discerning and interpreting the sounds of interest in the context of multiple simultaneous auditory stimuli (e.g., having a conversation while there is background noise, locating where sounds are coming from) can be attributed to both central and peripheral etiologies.

Alternative hearing difficulties are worth considering. For instance patients with dementia with Lewy bodies may report hearing muffled voices or a continuous musical tune if not overt auditory hallucinations (Golden and Josephs, 2015). However, patients with isolated hearing impairment may also experience auditory hallucinations, often of complex nature, which they recognize as unreal. Patients with frontotemporal dementia may develop aversion from or interest in particular sounds (including musicophilia) (Fletcher et al., 2015).

Ancillary investigations include audiometry and brainstem auditory evoked potentials. In cases were sensory hearing loss is detected, cognitive evaluation should rely less on auditory functions and more on visual abilities. In addition, evaluation of the etiology of the hearing loss and its treatment by a specialist is encouraged.

Diagnosis: Alzheimer disease masquerading as hearing impairment

Tip: Auditory function must be evaluated and treated in the context of cognitive impairment. Discerning between deficits in sound detection and auditory cognition is useful from diagnostic and treatment perspectives.

References

Campbell, J. and Sharma, A. 2013. Compensatory changes in cortical resource allocation in adults with hearing loss. *Front Syst Neurosci* **7** 71.

Deal, J. A. et al. 2017. Hearing impairment and incident dementia and cognitive decline in older adults: the health ABC study. *J Gerontol A Biol Sci Med Sci* **72**(5) 703–709.

Fletcher, P. D. et al. 2015. Auditory hedonic phenotypes in dementia: a behavioural and neuroanatomical analysis. *Cortex* **67** 95–105.

Golden, E. C. and Josephs, K. A. 2015. Minds on replay: musical hallucinations and their relationship to neurological disease. *Brain* **138**(Pt 12) 3793–3802.

Hardy, C. J. et al. 2016. Hearing and dementia. *J Neurol* **263** (11) 2339–2354.

Jayakody, D. M. P., Friedland, P. L., Martins, R. N. and Sohrabi, H. R. 2018. Impact of aging on the auditory system and related cognitive functions: a narrative review. *Front Neurosci* **12** 125.

Lin, F. R. et al. 2011. Hearing loss and cognition in the Baltimore Longitudinal Study of Aging. *Neuropsychology* **25** (6) 763–770.

Wingfield, A. et al. 2006. Effects of adult aging and hearing loss on comprehension of rapid speech varying in syntactic complexity. *J Am Acad Audiol* **17**(7) 487–497.

Case: This 58-year-old right-handed man presented with a 1-year history of personality changes. Previously characterized as being a serious and taciturn man, he was now extroverted, approaching and talking to strangers. Although he would show affection to others, and hugged often, his wife described him as being more emotionally distant from her. He started to deliver jokes as puns, something he had never done before. Although he continued to dress and groom properly, he did not seem to pay the same attention to detail as he did before. He resumed smoking cigarettes, which he had quit 30 years ago. While he continued to run his glass business appropriately, his son, who worked with him, noted he was more generous than usual. There were neither issues with memory or language nor any concerns about cognition or mood.

During his otherwise unremarkable examination, he exhibited a cheerful mood with occasional simple jokes, which did not seem inappropriate. Montreal Cognitive Assessment (MoCA) score was 30/30. Neuropsychological evaluation, including executive abilities testing, was within normal limits. Brain MRI was also reported as unremarkable.

Does a Normal Neuropsychological Evaluation Rule Out Neurocognitive Abnormalities?

The change in personality characterized by the development of excessive jocularity, also known as *Witzelsucht*, with some degree of personal neglect, impulsivity, and hyperorality (i.e., resuming smoking after 30 years) suggested an orbitofrontal syndrome. These changes, in the context of absent empathy, met the criteria for the diagnosis of behavioral variant of frontotemporal dementia (bvFTD) (see Case 7) (Rascovsky et al., 2011).

Neuropsychological evaluations compare the performance of a subject with normative data, typically obtained from a large, randomly selected sample from the wider representative population. Expected test performances are usually adjusted according to variables like age, sex, and education. However, focusing on whether the performance in a certain test is within a normal range or not will divert attention from assessing a change in cognition or behavior, which is more relevant in the assessment of neurodegenerative disorders. Even assessing decline can be challenging on the first evaluation as predicting premorbid performance is difficult (Duff, 2010). A "false normal" neuropsychological evaluation can result from a higher cognitive baseline, the ability to compensate, or an incomplete assessment of the cognitive domains affected. In this case, there was a clear history of behavioral changes in a highly educated subject (he had 22 years of formal education), sufficient to suspect the initial stage of a neurodegenerative process.

Doesn't Executive Abilities Testing Evaluate the Integrity of the Prefrontal Cortex?

Although the terms *prefrontal* and *executive abilities* are usually used interchangeably, they are not identical in meaning. First, not all executive abilities rely solely on prefrontal cortex integrity (Bettcher et al., 2016). Second, in addition to executive abilities, the prefrontal lobes are involved in cognitive and social-emotional processes. Finally, executive abilities tests are more sensitive to lateral prefrontal cortex–based function (Table 4.1), which is usually affected later in the course of bvFTD rather than orbitofrontal-based functions, which are usually affected early in the disease (Gregory et al., 1999; Krueger et al., 2011). Therefore, behavioral changes usually present before cognitive deficits can be documented on bedside testing.

An FDG-PET scan showed hypometabolism in the orbitofrontal cortex, right greater than left (Figure 4.1), supporting the diagnosis of bvFTD.

Discussion

Understanding the role of the prefrontal cortex (PFC) in cognition and behavior remains a challenge. Although there is a consensus that the PFC participates in higher-order functions, which include executive abilities, there is no agreement on the definition of these abilities. In addition, although the basis of cognitive function has traditionally been attributed to discrete cortical regions, we now understand them as contingent on the connectivity of large-scale networks

Table 4.1 Prefrontal cortex regions with associated lesion-related symptoms and suggested assessments

Region	Symptoms when affected	Formal assessment
Superior medial prefrontal– cingulate cortex	• Lack of initiative • Apathy • Abulia	Apathy evaluation scale Neuropsychiatric inventory – apathy section
Lateral prefrontal cortex	• Short-term (working) memory deficits • Difficulties in multitasking • Lack of organization, planning, or problem solving	Backward digit span Luria sequence Go/no-go Trail making test B Phonemic/design fluency Clock drawing
Orbitofrontal cortex	• Disinhibition • Emotional dysregulation (e.g., lability, irritability) • Altered social cognition and behavior (e.g., puerility, inappropriate and informal behavior) • Environmental dependency (e.g., echolalia, stimulus boundness, constant manipulation of objects) • Altered food habits (e.g., food fads, hyperphagia)	Neuropsychiatric inventory Frontal behavioral inventory
Frontopolar cortex	• Self-awareness • Impaired theory of mind • Loss of empathy	Sally-Anne test "Reading the mind in the eye" test

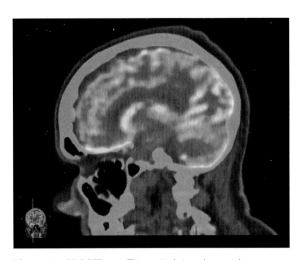

Figure 4.1 FDG-PET scan. This sagittal view shows right orbitofrontal hypometabolism. For the colour version, please refer to the plate section.

in the nervous system (Mesulam, 1998). In the case of the PFC, the most accepted model proposes parallel prefrontal-thalamic-pallido-striatal networks, which are involved in the different cognitive and behavioral functions attributed to the PFC (Alexander et al., 1986). This suggests that damage anywhere in the network may lead to similar deficits as focal PFC injury.

Currently, the most accepted parcellation of the PFC divides it into four functional areas (Table 4.1). Beyond the widely recognized (though loosely defined) executive abilities, damage to specific regions in the PFC may lead to changes in behavior and social cognition undetected by formal cognitive testing. Impairment in the orbitofrontal cortex, as in this case, is a good example. Careful history from the patient and informants is crucial for its detection. Appropriately sensitive questionnaires, like the Neuropsychiatric Inventory (NPI) Frontal Behavioral Inventory (FBI), and Frontal Systems Behavioral Scale (FrSBe) should be considered (Cummings, 1997; Kertesz et al., 1997). In addition, damage to medial prefrontal and cingulate cortex can lead to decreased initiative and drive. These patients consistently perform tasks appropriately but slowly, usually running out of time before completion. They should also be assessed with the NPI and Apathy Evaluation Scale (Marin et al., 1991). Finally, damage to the frontal poles may affect self-awareness and the ability to infer other people's thoughts and feelings, known as theory of mind. Identifying these changes in behavior are crucial as they precede detectable cognitive change in bvFTD by many years (Gregory et al., 1999).

Diagnosis: Possible behavioral variant of frontotemporal dementia

Tip: A normal neuropsychological evaluation does not preclude the diagnosis of an early neurodegenerative dementia syndrome in the context of progressive behavioral changes. Both should be thoroughly investigated with more sensitive scales, as they may represent early bvFTD.

References

Alexander, G. E., DeLong, M. R. and Strick, P. L. 1986. Parallel organization of functionally segregated circuits linking basal ganglia and cortex. *Annu Rev Neurosci* **9** 357–381.

Bettcher, B. M. et al. 2016. Neuroanatomical substrates of executive functions: beyond prefrontal structures. *Neuropsychologia* **85** 100–109.

Cummings, J. L. 1997. The Neuropsychiatric Inventory: assessing psychopathology in dementia patients. *Neurology* **48**(5 Suppl 6) S10–16.

Duff, K. 2010. Predicting premorbid memory functioning in older adults. *Appl Neuropsychol* **17**(4) 278–282.

Gregory, C. A., Serra-Mestres, J. and Hodges, J. R. 1999. Early diagnosis of the frontal variant of frontotemporal dementia: how sensitive are standard neuroimaging and neuropsychologic tests? *Neuropsychiatry Neuropsychol Behav Neurol* **12**(2) 128–135.

Kertesz, A., Davidson, W. and Fox, H. 1997. Frontal behavioral inventory: diagnostic criteria for frontal lobe dementia. *Can J Neurol Sci* **24**(1) 29–36.

Krueger, C. E. et al. 2011. Double dissociation in the anatomy of socioemotional disinhibition and executive functioning in dementia. *Neuropsychology* **25**(2) 249–259.

Marin, R. S., Biedrzycki, R. C. and Firinciogullari, S. 1991. Reliability and validity of the Apathy Evaluation Scale. *Psychiatry Res* **38**(2) 143–162.

Mesulam, M. M. 1998. From sensation to cognition. *Brain* **121**(6) 1013–1052.

Rascovsky, K. et al. 2011. Sensitivity of revised diagnostic criteria for the behavioural variant of frontotemporal dementia. *Brain* **134**(Pt 9) 2456–2477.

Case: This 80-year-old woman presented with a 5-year history of cognitive and behavioral changes. She first experienced depressed mood along with diminished interest in social activities. Around the same time, her daughter noticed that she relied on copious written notes to track information and intermittently seemed confused, affecting her ability to navigate familiar routes. A formal neuropsychological evaluation showed mild cognitive impairment (MCI) of the frontal-subcortical type (i.e., nonamnestic MCI). Routine lab work and brain MRI were reported as normal. Evaluation by a psychiatrist suggested a diagnosis of acute depression in the context of litigation involving her son and the family business. Cognitive changes were attributed to depression (Alexopoulos et al., 2002).

She was treated with multiple medications, including buspirone, sertraline, and bupropion. In addition, she underwent cognitive behavioral therapy. Her therapist noted a flat affect and monotone voice. She did not endorse depression but became increasingly withdrawn, and her difficulties with work routine prompted her retirement from the family business. A full-time caregiver was hired for cooking and housecleaning. Driving privileges were removed because of inattention and poor concentration.

Repeat neuropsychological evaluation, 13 months after the first one was reported as unchanged, indicating her preserved ability to learn and recall new material. However, her performance was marked by confabulatory tendencies and irrelevant responses (e.g., intrusions and perseverations). Ratings on the Beck Depression Inventory (BDI) did not suggest depression. Given the stability of her cognitive performance, depression was considered as the main cause of her decline. She was not thought to have a neurodegenerative dementia. Methylphenidate and memantine were prescribed, reportedly to help with her level of energy, mood, and cognition. However, she continued to decline. Her daughter complained that she had become very dependent on others. She would spend most of her day either in bed or watching TV, rarely getting up unless she was told to. Previously extroverted and social, she was now seldom interacting with people. She started eating impulsively, particularly at night, which resulted in weight gain.

On exam, she exhibited restricted and inappropriately elevated affect (moria), reduced spontaneous gesture, and monoprosodic voice without hypophonia. She didn't speak unless spoken to. Her comments were terse, concrete, and, although grammatically correct, simplified. At times her answers were impulsive, responding "yes" when she meant to say "no" or substituting habit phrases for answers ("definitely"). Intermittently her responses were echolalic, and if given a choice of two items, she would always choose the last one offered. Her description of the cookie theft picture was detailed and coherent, without hesitations, word-finding difficulties, paraphasias, or grammatical errors. Motor examination revealed slow tapping speed without decrement, rigidity and asymmetrical tremor affecting predominantly the right side. Intermittently, she patted her face with her hand or licked her lips. Gait was wide based with slow and decreased stride.

Given the Lack of Change in Her Neuropsychological Evaluation and the Prominent Behavioral Changes, Should We Consider This a Primary Psychiatric Condition?

Even without progressive cognitive impairment, changes in mood and behavior in individuals above the age 50 years may signal neurodegeneration. This has been termed mild behavioral impairment (MBI) (Box 5.1) (Ismail et al., 2016). In the presence of MCI, neuropsychiatric symptoms (NPS) are associated with poorer function and quality of life and greater annual risk for conversion to dementia (Feldman et al., 2004). Behavioral changes are well known to be initial symptoms of frontotemporal lobar degeneration but may also appear early on in the course in Alzheimer, Lewy body, and vascular diseases (Taragano et al., 2009). Failure to identify neurodegenerative etiologies for changes in mood or behavior leads, as in this case, to inappropriate medical treatment.

In this case, it seems the depressive symptoms were not significant as she did not endorse active depressive symptoms in the evaluation or on the BDI. However, the utility of the BDI is limited and more comprehensive behavioral evaluation is needed. Withdrawal and lack of initiative were more likely associated with apathy, which not uncommonly co-occur with depression, particularly in the context of a neurodegenerative process.

A Neuropsychiatric Inventory Questionnaire (NPI-Q) was administered to her family, revealing apathy, disinhibition, and abnormal motor behaviors. Other abnormal behaviors reported included hoarding and lack of care for her personal appearance, uncommon for someone who had always been very attentive to her weight and appearance. She was eating excessively and continuously, until she vomited, and now favored potatoes as her food of choice.

CSF biomarkers for Alzheimer disease were negative. A [18F] fluorodeoxyglucose (FDG)-PET scan revealed bilateral hypometabolism in the frontal and temporal lobes, worse on the left, and in the anterior parietal lobe and left thalamus, suggestive of frontotemporal lobar degeneration. Given the presence of apathy, disinhibition, ritualistic behavior and changes in food preferences, in the context of frontotemporal hypometabolism, she was diagnosed with probable behavioral variant of frontotemporal dementia (bvFTD).

Should We Consider Further Management of Her Depression?

The presence of depression increases disability and dependency, lowers quality of life, and accelerates decline in patients with cognitive impairment (Black and Almeida, 2004; Rapp et al., 2011). At least 25 percent of individuals with Alzheimer disease will develop depression symptoms (Starkstein et al., 2011). Depression rates are even higher in dementia with Lewy bodies and frontotemporal dementia (Ballard et al., 2004; Chakrabarty et al., 2015). Multiple risk factors contribute to depression: personal and family history of depression, increasing age, female sex, severity and duration of dementia, impaired communication, medical comorbidities, impaired insight, and a premorbid neurotic personality (Ford, 2014). Treatment of depression is challenging. Approximately 30 percent of individuals will have limited if any response to treatment, even with changes in drug regimens. The chance of a successful drug trial is halved with each subsequent medication (Rush et al., 2006). In the context of cognitive impairment, there is even less evidence to

guide management. While some individual studies support the use of antidepressants, particularly SSRIs for mood impairment in the context of depression, some meta-analyses question the long-term benefit of antidepressants in dementia (Dudas et al., 2018). Interestingly, donepezil and memantine have been shown to improve behavior (Cummings et al., 2016; McShane et al., 2006). Although the quality of individual studies varies, modest benefits may be accrued from psychological therapies, including cognitive behavioral therapy (CBT), interpersonal therapy and counseling (Orgeta et al., 2014).

Discussion

Depression used to be considered an independent cause of cognitive and functional decline but is now considered a manifestation of neuropathological changes and possibly the presenting, or prodromal, symptom of a neurodegenerative disease. Most commonly, depression and irritability with milder degrees of apathy are associated with Alzheimer disease pathology. It is now clear that a wide range of changes in mood and behavior can be the presenting symptom of neurodegenerative diseases (Ismail et al., 2018). Simply screening for depression will miss other behavioral abnormalities and mood disturbances. Late-onset depression associated with anxiety can be indicative of an alpha-synucleinopathy (Goldman and Postuma, 2014). Psychotic symptoms consisting of early well-developed delusions, visual hallucinations, and a sense of presence are also common across the Lewy body diseases, namely, Parkinson disease, Parkinson disease dementia, and dementia with Lewy bodies. In Alzheimer disease, delusions usually are accusations of theft or infidelity and occur mid-stage well after significant memory and other cognitive symptoms. Marked apathy, disinhibition, abnormal motor movements, and loss of empathy are suggestive of frontotemporal lobe degeneration pathology, including tau, TDP-43, and FUS. As in this case, behavior changes are often the most remarkable features of frontotemporal dementias. Relying exclusively on cognitive test results will miss the diagnosis.

The measurement of neuropsychiatric symptoms is often dismissed when cognitive or primary psychiatric disorders are the focus of concern. Even common NPS scales, such as the NPI-Q or Frontal Behavioral Inventory (FBI), center on dementia-stage symptoms and miss crucial early behavioral signs of neurodegenerative disease in preclinical, prodromal, subjective cognitive impairment or early mild cognitive

---

Box 5.1 Mild Behavioral Impairment Criteria

1. Changes in behavior or personality observed by patient or informant or clinician, starting later in life (age $\geq$ 50) and persisting at least intermittently for $\geq$6 months. These represent clear change from the person's usual behavior or personality as evidenced by at least one of the following:
   a. Decreased motivation (e.g., apathy, aspontaneity, indifference)
   b. Affective dysregulation (e.g., anxiety, dysphoria, changeability, euphoria, irritability)
   c. Impulse dyscontrol (e.g., agitation, disinhibition, gambling, obsessiveness, behavioral perseveration, stimulus bind)
   d. Social inappropriateness (e.g., lack of empathy, loss of insight, loss of social graces or tact, rigidity, exaggeration of previous personality traits)
   e. Abnormal perception or thought content (e.g., delusions, hallucinations)
2. Behaviors are of sufficient severity to produce at least minimal impairment in at least one of the following areas:
   a. Interpersonal relationships
   b. Other aspects of social functioning
   c. Ability to perform in the workplace
3. The patient should generally maintain his/her independence of function in daily life, with minimal aids or assistance.
4. Although comorbid conditions may be present, the behavioral or personality changes are not attributable to another current psychiatric disorder (e.g., generalized anxiety disorder, major depression, manic or psychotic disorders), traumatic or general medical causes, or the physiological effects of a substance or medication.
5. The patient does not meet criteria for a dementia syndrome (e.g., Alzheimer dementia, frontotemporal dementia, dementia with Lewy bodies, vascular dementia, other dementia). Mild cognitive impairment (MCI) can be concurrently diagnosed with mild behavioral impairment.

---

impairment stages. An MBI-specific rating scale, the MBI checklist (MBI-C, freely available at www.MBItest.org), is based on the ISTAART-AA MBI criteria (Ismail et al., 2017). The goal of the MBI-C is to assist in the assessment of late-life NPS. This 34-question informant-rated questionnaire probes domains of apathy, emotional dysregulation, impulsivity and agitation, social cognition, and psychosis.

Diagnosis: Behavioral variant frontotemporal dementia evolving into corticobasal syndrome (pathology undetermined)

Tip: Neurodegenerative disease may present with behavioral impairment preceding cognitive decline. Depression or progressive behavioral changes (including apathy, eating disorders, and impulse control disorders) presenting after the age of 50 years should raise the concern for neurodegenerative disorders, even when cognitive screening is normal. Ascertainment of mild behavioral impairment requires behavioral screen tools such as the NPI-Q, FBI, or MBI. Finally, a clue that depression may not be the driver of behavioral changes is its unresponsiveness to standard antidepressants.

References

Alexopoulos, G. S. et al. 2002. Clinical presentation of the "depression-executive dysfunction syndrome" of late life. *Am J Geriatr Psychiatry* **10**(1) 98–106.

Ballard, C. G. et al. 2004. Neuropathological substrates of psychiatric symptoms in prospectively studied patients with autopsy-confirmed dementia with Lewy bodies. *Am J Psychiatry* **161**(5) 843–849.

Black, W. and Almeida, O. P. 2004. A systematic review of the association between the behavioral and psychological symptoms of dementia and burden of care. *Int Psychogeriatr* **16**(3) 295–315.

Chakrabarty, T., Sepehry, A. A., Jacova, C. and Hsiung, G. Y. 2015. The prevalence of depressive symptoms in frontotemporal dementia: a meta-analysis. *Dement Geriatr Cogn Disord* **39**(5–6) 257–271.

Cummings, J. et al. 2016. Role of donepezil in the management of neuropsychiatric symptoms in Alzheimer's disease and dementia with Lewy bodies. *CNS Neurosci Ther* **22**(3) 159–166.

Dudas, R., Malouf, R., McCleery, J. and Dening, T. 2018. Antidepressants for treating depression in dementia. *Cochrane Database Syst Rev* **8** Cd003944.

Feldman, H. et al. 2004. Behavioral symptoms in mild cognitive impairment. *Neurology* **62**(7) 1199–1201.

Ford, A. H. 2014. Neuropsychiatric aspects of dementia. *Maturitas* **79**(2) 209–215.

Goldman, J. G. and Postuma, R. 2014. Premotor and nonmotor features of Parkinson's disease. *Curr Opin Neurol* **27**(4) 434–441.

Ismail, Z. et al. 2016. Neuropsychiatric symptoms as early manifestations of emergent dementia: provisional diagnostic criteria for mild behavioral impairment. *Alzheimers Dement* **12**(2) 195–202.

Ismail, Z. et al. 2017. The Mild Behavioral Impairment Checklist (MBI-C): a rating scale for neuropsychiatric symptoms in pre-dementia populations. *J Alzheimers Dis* **56**(3) 929–938.

Ismail, Z. et al. 2018. Affective and emotional dysregulation as pre-dementia risk markers: exploring the mild behavioral impairment symptoms of depression, anxiety, irritability, and euphoria. *Int Psychogeriatr* **30**(2) 185–196.

McShane, R., Areosa Sastre, A. and Minakaran, N. 2006. Memantine for dementia. *Cochrane Database Syst Rev* **2** Cd003154.

Orgeta, V., Qazi, A., Spector, A. E. and Orrell, M. 2014. Psychological treatments for depression and anxiety in dementia and mild cognitive impairment. *Cochrane Database Syst Rev* **1** Cd009125.

Rapp, M. A. et al. 2011. Cognitive decline in patients with dementia as a function of depression. *Am J Geriatr Psychiatry* **19**(4) 357–363.

Rush, A. J. et al. 2006. Bupropion-SR, sertraline, or venlafaxine-XR after failure of SSRIs for depression. *N Engl J Med* **354**(12) 1231–1242.

Starkstein, S. E. et al. 2011. Diagnostic criteria for depression in Alzheimer disease: a study of symptom patterns using latent class analysis. *Am J Geriatr Psychiatry* **19**(6) 551–558.

Taragano, F. E. et al. 2009. Mild behavioral impairment and risk of dementia: a prospective cohort study of 358 patients. *J Clin Psychiatry* **70**(4) 584–592.

CASE

6 "The Thing about Remembering Names of Things"

Case: This 63-year-old right-handed woman presented with a 4-year history of "memory" decline. Her husband first became concerned when in a response to a text message that he sent notifying her that he had arranged transportation for her father's medical visits, she responded, "Great, but what does transportation mean?" Her vocabulary became progressively simpler and less specific (e.g., dog or animal for bulldog), and later she substituted the word "thing" for almost any noun. More recently, she increasingly asked for the name and function of common objects (e.g., screwdriver). She repetitively interjected stereotyped phrases (e.g., "you have to be happy, happy, and happy") that were often unrelated to the topic or emotional tone of the discussion. Previously an avid reader of a wide variety of fiction and nonfiction books, her current choices were from the children's section of the library. Her husband now had to schedule their activities around her desire to be home each day to watch *The Muppet Show*. Despite her impairments, she continued to be spontaneously verbal and would inappropriately approach strangers to engage in a conversation. Within the past year she had developed the habit of collecting random papers. Her interest in foods changed frequently and were often constrained to one or two items at a time.

On exam, she exhibited moria (i.e., childish jocularity), even as she described her memory difficulties. In the interview, spontaneous speech was fluent without hesitations, and there were no deficits in prosody, volume, articulation, or cadence. Her comments were often tangential, and she lapsed into a perseverative discussion of her enjoyment of *The Muppet Show* characters. The cognitive evaluation revealed impairments in executive function (backward digit span, clock drawing and trails B), learning (from a list of 10 words, she learned 5, freely recalled 4 and later recognized the same 4 from a list), and language (could only name 5 objects from a list of 15), and phonemic and semantic fluencies (4 and 7 over one minute, respectively). The remainder of her neurological examination was unremarkable.

Does She Have a Memory Impairment?

In clinical practice, memory complaints usually refer to impairments in declarative memory (i.e., memories that can be consciously recalled). Two memory systems have been described in declarative memory: episodic (EM) and semantic memory (SM). EM includes recollections of personal previous experiences placed in a time and space context. Semantic memory refers to general knowledge of facts and concepts regarding the world, not located in a specific time or place. While EM impairment is one of the first relevant features of Alzheimer disease, isolated impairment in SM is one of the early features of semantic dementia (SD). Impairments in SM may be erroneously misattributed to EM deficits, so differentiating between them has diagnostic relevance (Table 6.1).

SD represents an associative agnosia affecting multiple cognitive domains beyond language (Hodges and Patterson, 2007). However, in recent years SD has been included as a semantic variant of primary progressive aphasia (svPPA) and its clinical criteria has been limited to impairments in language (Gorno-Tempini et al., 2011). This may lead to an incomplete assessment due to a disregard of the evaluation of other potentially affected domains (e.g., visual association). With this caveat in mind, we will refer to SD as svPPA, given that this is the common usage in the current literature.

It should be noted that on her evaluation, she could only recall 4 out of the 10 words. However, she was only able to learn five in the first place, suggesting learning impairment rather than an isolated EM disorder. Moreover, on comprehensive language evaluation, our patient exhibited impaired naming, single-word comprehension, object knowledge, and surface dyslexia, with normal repetition and fluency (Video 6.1), meeting criteria for svPPA (Table 6.2) (Gorno-Tempini et al., 2011). A brain MRI showed asymmetric anterior

Video 6.1 The examination demonstrates normal fluency and grammar. Anomia and language simplification with the use of supraordinates ("animal" or "dog" instead of "lion") are observed when asked to describe a series of pictures. Anomia and lack of knowledge of the function of objects are also noted when shown different pictures. Surface dyslexia and lack of single-word comprehension becomes evident when asked to read a paragraph. Through the video, the patient exhibits childish jocularity.

Table 6.1 Episodic and semantic memory distinguishing features

Characteristic	Episodic memory	Semantic memory
Type of memories	Events, episodes	Facts, ideas, concepts
Organization	Chronological	Conceptual
Report	"I remember"	"I know"
Example	Remembering what you had for dinner	Knowing the capital of Argentina
Evaluation	Tests of recall and recognition	Test including naming and object knowledge
Major anatomical areas[a]	Medial temporal lobe	Anterior temporal lobe

[a] Recent evidence has raised doubt about whether episodic and semantic memory systems are separate networks, proposing instead that they rely on partially overlapping large-scale brain networks that include not only the medial and lateral temporal lobes but also portions of the frontal and parietal lobes.

Table 6.2 Diagnostic criteria for the semantic variant of primary progressive aphasia (svPPA)

Clinical diagnosis of svPPA

Both of the following core features must be present:

1. Impaired confrontation naming
2. Impaired single-word comprehension

At least 3 of the following other diagnostic features must be present:

1. Impaired object knowledge, particularly for low-frequency or low-familiarity items
2. Surface dyslexia or dysgraphia
3. Spared repetition
4. Spared speech production (grammar and motor speech)

Imaging-supported semantic variant PPA diagnosis

Both of the following criteria must be present:

1. Clinical diagnosis of svPPA
2. Imaging must show one or more of the following results:
   a. Predominant anterior temporal lobe atrophy
   b. Predominant anterior temporal hypoperfusion or hypometabolism on SPECT or PET

Source: Gorno-Tempini et al. (2011).

temporal atrophy (Figure 6.1) further supporting the clinical diagnosis.

Should the Diagnosis of Behavioral Variant of Frontotemporal Dementia (bvFTD) Be Considered?

Her progressive behavioral changes (i.e., disinhibition, compulsive behaviors, dietary changes, and executive deficits) fit criteria for bvFTD. However, language was the first domain affected, and therefore primary progressive aphasia should be considered first. Behavioral changes should not exclude the

diagnosis of PPA as they are usually observed in the course of svPPA.

Is It Relevant to Distinguish between bvFTD and svPPA?

While up to half of bvFTD is familial, pure svPPA is rarely so (Rohrer et al., 2009). Therefore, pursuing genetic testing may be warranted only for bvFTD cases to fulfill the objectives of securing a final etiology, assist in prognostication, and make genetic counseling available to the patient and the family. Management may also differ between these disorders, since communication strategies are important in svPPA, but behavioral modifications may apply more to bvFTD. Finally, from a neuropathology perspective, the vast majority of svPPA patients exhibit TDP-43 type C pathology, while bvFTD is associated with either tau, TDP-43 (pathology types A, B, and D), or fused in sarcoma (FUS) pathology among others (Mann and Snowden, 2017).

Discussion

The svPPA syndrome is associated with early degeneration of the anterior temporal pole (ATL), which serves as a hub for semantic memory (Patterson et al., 2007). Early involvement of the left (dominant) ATL is more frequent in svPPA and presents with semantic language impairment, while the right (nondominant) ATL, if involved first, with behavioral changes and prosopagnosia (see Case 14) (Thompson et al., 2003). Initially unilateral, ATL pathology eventually spreads contralaterally.

Patients typically exhibit word-finding and single-word comprehension difficulties at the onset. Speech is fluent, without the prolonged word-finding pauses seen

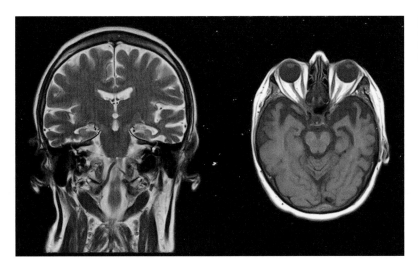

Figure 6.1 T2 coronal and T1 axial brain MRI in this patient. Note the bilateral anterior temporal atrophy, more pronounced on the left.

in other PPA variants, but empty, with frequent circumlocutions, simplifications, and semantic paraphasias (Rohrer et al., 2008). As the disease progresses, object knowledge is lost with inability to recall or recognize object name and function, without benefit from cueing (Karageorgiou and Miller, 2014). Surface dyslexia, defined as the inability to read irregular words correctly (e.g., colonel, yacht), is also observed. Executive function and visuospatial skills typically are preserved early in the course. As the disease spreads from the temporal lobes to the prefrontal cortex behavioral changes occur, such as irritability, perseveration, apathy, and loss of empathy (Bang et al., 2015). During late stages, most patients become essentially mute, with only a limited repertoire of stereotypic phrases and a complete loss of word comprehension (Landin-Romero et al., 2016).

Structural imaging reveals bilateral but asymmetric atrophy of the anterior temporal lobes, most often left lateralized, with later atrophy in the inferior frontal region. Functional neuroimaging studies show a similar pattern of hypometabolism. These findings serve as supportive for svPPA (Landin-Romero et al., 2016).

Diagnosis: Semantic dementia (SD) or semantic variant of primary progressive aphasia (svPPA)

Tip: When presented with memory complaints, distinction between episodic and semantic memory impairment is of key importance. While behavioral abnormalities may suggest a behavioral variant of FTD, the early appearance and sustained prominence of anomia and loss of semantic knowledge means svPPA should be given precedence in the differential

diagnosis. When svPPA is suspected, other domains beyond language should be evaluated.

References

Bang, J., Spina, S. and Miller, B. L. 2015. Frontotemporal dementia. *Lancet* **386**(10004) 1672–1682.

Gorno-Tempini, M. L. et al. 2011. Classification of primary progressive aphasia and its variants. *Neurology* **76**(11) 1006–1014.

Hodges, J. R. and Patterson, K. 2007. Semantic dementia: a unique clinicopathological syndrome. *Lancet Neurol* **6**(11) 1004–1014.

Karageorgiou, E. and Miller, B. L. 2014. Frontotemporal lobar degeneration: a clinical approach. *Semin Neurol* **34**(2) 189–201.

Landin-Romero, R., Tan, R., Hodges, J. R. and Kumfor, F. 2016. An update on semantic dementia: genetics, imaging, and pathology. *Alzheimers Res Ther* **8**(1) 52.

Mann, D. M. A. and Snowden, J. S. 2017. Frontotemporal lobar degeneration: pathogenesis, pathology and pathways to phenotype. *Brain Pathol* **27**(6) 723–736.

Patterson, K., Nestor, P. J. and Rogers, T. T. 2007. Where do you know what you know? The representation of semantic knowledge in the human brain. *Nat Rev Neurosci* **8**(12) 976–987.

Rohrer, J. D. et al. 2008. Word-finding difficulty: a clinical analysis of the progressive aphasias. *Brain* **131**(Pt 1) 8–38.

Rohrer, J. D. et al. 2009. The heritability and genetics of frontotemporal lobar degeneration. *Neurology* **73**(18) 1451–1456.

Thompson, S. A., Patterson, K. and Hodges, J. R. 2003. Left/right asymmetry of atrophy in semantic dementia: behavioral-cognitive implications. *Neurology* **61**(9) 1196–1203.

Case: Over the last 18 months, this 72-year-old woman developed memory difficulties. She forgot requests made within hours, repeated queries multiple times during the day regarding the date, and could not learn how to operate new tools. She appeared largely unaware of her cognitive deficits. Her husband denied changes in language or personality. Her deceased mother had unspecified problems with memory in her late seventies. Of her seven sisters, one had problems with language presenting in her early sixties, another word-finding difficulty was noticed in her late sixties, and a third had presumed Parkinson disease without apparent cognitive impairment manifesting during her mid-fifties. On exam she was alert and fully oriented. Her conversational speech was fluent and she was able to follow commands (Video 7.1). Montreal Cognitive Assessment (MoCA) score was 14/30 with impairments in attention, naming, phonemic fluency, abstraction, and delayed recall (she was unable to recall any words freely, but recognized 2 out of 5 words when multiple choices were given). The remainder of her examination was remarkable only for mild mirror movements and stimulus-sensitive axial myoclonus, expressed as excessive startle. A diagnosis of familial Alzheimer disease (AD) was made, and she was started on donepezil.

Are Her Deficits and Family History Sufficient to Suspect a Genetic Form of Alzheimer Disease?

Although her chief complaint was memory decline, MoCA screening demonstrated impairments in other domains too, including attention. Performance on all aspects of cognitive testing can be greatly affected by attentional deficits. In addition the heterogeneity of cognitive impairments in her family history plus a family history of Parkinson disease should make the tentative diagnosis of AD suspect.

How Should We Evaluate This Patient?

Because of the history of heterogeneous phenotypes in the family, and the evidence of attentional deficits in her initial visit, further investigation of the frontally mediated cognitive and behavioral domains should be done. Behavior should not be solely assessed with the information collected during the interview but also evaluated through objective, standardized instruments. Thus, the husband was presented with the Frontal Behavioral Inventory (FBI), a caregiver-centered questionnaire aimed to identify the presence and severity of changes in behaviors and personality. The score ranges from 0 to 72, with higher scores representing more impairment and scores above 27 are considered abnormal. Her total score was 13. However, through this instrument it became clear that the patient manifested moderate apathy, lack of spontaneity, and disorganization, with mild inflexibility, personal neglect, inattention, logopenia, and loss of insight, plus mild disinhibition with irritability and hoarding. Further inquiry revealed that these changes in behavior presented before any difficulties with memory had occurred. A modified Consortium to Establish a Registry for Alzheimer's Disease (CERAD) battery revealed a variable rate of learning (she recalled five words on the first trial, seven on the second, and six on the third), further suggesting the effects of impaired attention and concentration on learning. She was unable to freely recall any of the words later. However, her performance on recognition suggested better encoding and retention of learned material than was demonstrated by her responses without cues. Her language evaluation was remarkable for impaired verbal fluency. Her phonemic fluency, associated with left frontal networks and non-Alzheimer pathology, was significantly worse than her semantic fluency, associated with posterior networks and AD pathology. During the exam, she displayed elevated affect with childish jocularity, also referred to as moria, and was inappropriately informal, repeatedly asking when she was going to eat.

The frontal behaviors identified on FBI and seen on exam, the retrieval deficit in memory with signs of fluctuating attention affecting learning, and impaired phonemic rather than semantic fluency, align with frontally mediated pathologies and suggested a clinical

---

Video 7.1 The examination shows normal speech and motor evaluation. She appears to have limited insight to her deficits.

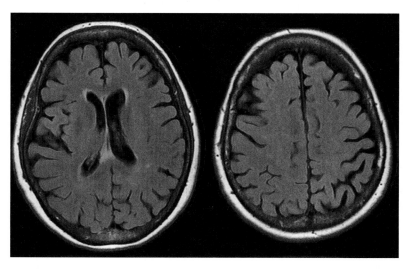

Figure 7.1 FLAIR axial brain MRI demonstrating asymmetric ventricular system with enlargement of the left anterior horn of the lateral ventricles, suggesting left-predominant frontal atrophy. Left-predominant parietal atrophy is evident in the higher axial view.

diagnosis of, behavioral variant frontotemporal dementia (bvFTD), rather than AD.

In support of this clinical diagnosis, the brain MRI showed an asymmetric ventricular system with enlargement of the left anterior horn of the lateral ventricles, indirectly suggesting left-predominant fronto-parietal atrophy (Figure 7.1).

How Was a Diagnosis Determined?

The evaluation of one of the patient's sisters met criteria for agrammatic variant of primary progressive aphasia, which had progressed to death within five years from symptom onset. Her autopsy showed changes consistent with frontotemporal lobar degeneration with TDP-43 type A proteinopathy. Blood progranulin levels were reduced. Genetic assessment of her progranulin gene (*GRN*) identified a pathogenic mutation. With this information, genetic analysis led to the confirmation of the same genetic disorder in our patient.

Discussion

When a patient complains of memory deficits and shows impaired recall in the clinic or at the bedside, the nature of associated impairments clarifies whether the amnestic syndrome is primary or secondary to other deficits or behaviors. The assessment of any cognitive domain depends to some extent on the patient's level of attention, defined as the ability to selectively process information in the environment. Anterograde episodic verbal memory, the feature of memory most commonly evaluated in the clinic, also depends of the patient's capacity to encode (form) the memory,

consolidate it, and then retrieve it (Budson, 2009). Although the mechanisms of episodic memory are insufficiently understood, there is wide agreement that the hippocampus and the medial temporal lobe play a critical role in the encoding and consolidation of memory, whereas the prefrontal cortex is highly active during the retrieval of episodic memories (Budson, 2009; Dickerson and Eichenbaum, 2010). Therefore, impaired memory performance due to defective encoding, secondary to a process affecting the temporal lobe, usually does not benefit from recognition. Conversely, patients with impaired memory retrieval, due to prefrontal dysfunction as often observed in Parkinson disease, are more likely to recognize information they could not recall freely (Hornberger et al., 2010).

The diagnosis of bvFTD is dependent on the identification of a progressive deterioration of personality, social behavior, and cognition (Table 7.1) (Rascovsky et al., 2011). Since these patients frequently have impaired insight into their deficits, informants are of major importance for the diagnosis (Mendez and Shapira, 2005). Initial changes in personality or behavior frequently go unrecognized. Even in cases where a change is noticed, this might be assumed as a normal "quirk" in the patient's personality or attributed to a psychiatric disorder (Pressman and Miller, 2014). In our case, the husband only described abnormal behaviors when asked through a formal instrument. Patients usually present to the neurology clinic once the cognitive deterioration is overt and widespread. Identification of early behavioral changes that would raise the possibility of bvFTD also has implication for genetic counseling, as up to 50 percent of bvFTD

Table 7.1 Diagnostic criteria for the behavioral variant of frontotemporal dementia from Rascovsky et al. (2011)

I.   Neurodegenerative disease; following symptom must be present to meet criteria for bvFTD
      A.   Shows progressive deterioration of behavior and/or cognition by observation or history (as provided by a knowledgeable informant)

II.   Possible bvFTD

      Three of the following behavioral/cognitive symptoms (A–F) must be present to meet criteria; ascertainment requires that symptoms be persistent or recurrent, rather than single or rare events
      A.   Early behavioral disinhibition [one of the following symptoms (A.1–A.3) must be present]:
           A.1. Socially inappropriate behavior
           A.2. Loss of manners or decorum
           A.3. Impulsive, rash, or careless actions
      B.   Early apathy or inertia [one of the following symptoms (B.1–B.2) must be present]:
           B.1. Apathy
           B.2. Inertia
      C.   Early loss of sympathy or empathy [one of the following symptoms (C.1–C.2) must be present]:
           C.1. Diminished response to other people's needs and feelings
           C.2. Diminished social interest, interrelatedness, or personal warmth
      D.   Early perseverative, stereotyped, or compulsive/ritualistic behavior [one of the following symptoms (D.1–D.3) must be present]:
           D.1. Simple repetitive movements
           D.2. Complex, compulsive, or ritualistic behaviors
           D.3. Stereotypy of speech
      E.   Hyperorality and dietary changes [one of the following symptoms (E.1–E.3) must be present]:
           E.1. Altered food preferences
           E.2. Binge eating, increased consumption of alcohol or cigarettes
           E.3. Oral exploration or consumption of inedible objects
      F.   Neuropsychological profile: executive/generation deficits with relative sparing of memory and visuospatial functions [all of the following symptoms (F.1–F.3) must be present]:
           F.1. Deficits in executive tasks
           F.2. Relative sparing of episodic memory
           F.3. Relative sparing of visuospatial skills

III. Probable bvFTD

      All of the following symptoms (A–C) must be present to meet criteria:
      A.   Meets criteria for possible bvFTD
      B.   Exhibits significant functional decline (by caregiver report or as evidenced by Clinical Dementia Rating Scale or Functional Activities Questionnaire scores)
      C.   Imaging results consistent with bvFTD [one of the following (C.1–C.2) must be present]:
           C.1. Frontal and/or anterior temporal atrophy on MRI or CT
           C.2. Frontal and/or anterior temporal hypoperfusion or hypometabolism on PET or SPECT

IV.   Behavioral variant FTD with definite FTLD pathology criterion A and either criterion B or C must be present to meet criteria
      A.   Meets criteria for possible or probable bvFTD
      B.   Histopathological evidence of FTLD on biopsy or at postmortem
      C.   Presence of a known pathogenic mutation

V.   Exclusionary criteria for bvFTD
      Criteria A and B must be answered negatively for any bvFTD diagnosis; criterion C can be positive for possible bvFTD but must be negative for probable bvFTD
      A.   Pattern of deficits is better accounted for by other nondegenerative nervous system or medical disorders
      B.   Behavioral disturbance is better accounted for by a psychiatric diagnosis
      C.   Biomarkers strongly indicative of Alzheimer disease or other neurodegenerative process

Note: As a general guideline, "early" refers to symptom presentation within the first three years.

patients have a positive family history (Seelaar et al., 2011).

GRN mutations account for up to 10 percent of all FTD patients and 22 percent of the familial FTDs (Seelaar et al., 2011). The most common clinical presentation is bvFTD with apathy as the dominant feature (Beck et al., 2008). However, *GRN* mutations are characterized by clinical heterogeneity, encompassing language impairment, visuospatial dysfunction, and apraxia (Le Ber et al., 2008). Episodic memory disorders are also frequent, sometimes leading to the diagnosis of amnestic mild cognitive impairment (MCI) or AD (Kelley et al., 2010). Phenotypical diversity is may be seen within families with the same mutation, as we observed in this case (Rademakers et al., 2007).

Certain MRI findings may be suggestive of a *GRN* mutation. Asymmetric brain atrophy (documented in our patient) and white matter involvement (not appreciated in this case), initially affecting the parietal region, appear to be more common in *GRN* mutation carriers compared with non-*PGRN* FTD cases (Agosta et al., 2015; Whitwell et al., 2012).

Diagnosis: Behavioral variant of frontotemporal dementia due to *GRN* mutation

Tip: The thorough assessment of "memory" problems should include consideration of whether encoding or retrieval mechanisms are involved, and whether learning is impaired secondary to an attentional impairment. Other important elements include a formal analysis of behavior, a detailed family history, and a critical evaluation of the brain MRI for frontal lobe atrophy, asymmetry, and white matter involvement. *GRN* mutations lead to clinical heterogeneous phenotypes, including ostensibly primary memory impairment, and may be listed in the differential diagnosis of patients with asymmetric parietal atrophy on MRI.

References

Agosta, F. et al. 2015. MRI signatures of the frontotemporal lobar degeneration continuum. *Hum Brain Mapp* **7** 2602–2614.

Beck, J. et al. 2008. A distinct clinical, neuropsychological and radiological phenotype is associated with progranulin gene mutations in a large UK series. *Brain* **131**(Pt 3) 706–720.

Budson, A. E. 2009. Understanding memory dysfunction. *Neurologist* **15**(2) 71–79.

Dickerson, B. C. and Eichenbaum, H. 2010. The episodic memory system: neurocircuitry and disorders. *Neuropsychopharmacology* **35**(1) 86–104.

Hornberger, M. et al. 2010. How preserved is episodic memory in behavioral variant frontotemporal dementia? *Neurology* **74**(6) 472–479.

Kelley, B. J. et al. 2010. Alzheimer disease–like phenotype associated with the c.154delA mutation in progranulin. *Arch Neurol* **67**(2) 171–177.

Le Ber, I. et al. 2008. Phenotype variability in progranulin mutation carriers: a clinical, neuropsychological, imaging and genetic study. *Brain* **131**(Pt 3) 732–746.

Mendez, M. F. and Shapira, J. S. 2005. Loss of insight and functional neuroimaging in frontotemporal dementia. *J Neuropsychiatry Clin Neurosci* **17**(3) 413–416.

Pressman, P. S. and Miller, B. L. 2014. Diagnosis and management of behavioral variant frontotemporal dementia. *Biol Psychiatry* **75**(7) 574–581.

Rademakers, R. et al. 2007. Phenotypic variability associated with progranulin haploinsufficiency in patients with the common 1477C–<T (Arg493X) mutation: an international initiative. *Lancet Neurol* **6**(10) 857–868.

Rascovsky, K. et al. 2011. Sensitivity of revised diagnostic criteria for the behavioural variant of frontotemporal dementia. *Brain* **134**(Pt 9) 2456–2477.

Seelaar, H. et al. 2011. Clinical, genetic and pathological heterogeneity of frontotemporal dementia: a review. *J Neurol Neurosurg Psychiatry* **82**(5) 476–486.

Whitwell, J. L. et al. 2012. Neuroimaging signatures of frontotemporal dementia genetics: C9ORF72, tau, progranulin and sporadics. *Brain* **135**(Pt 3) 794–806.

Case: This 73-year-old man presented with a six-month history of progressive cognitive and behavioral decline along with balance impairment. His family first noticed he had visual and auditory hallucinations, as he talked to imaginary people and seemed to be feeding imaginary birds. In addition, he started having problems with his balance, which led to several falls. In the following months, his memory and ability to communicate declined. His level of alertness fluctuated, and at times he was confused and unable to follow directions. Irritability emerged, manifested by frequent swaying of his arms in disdain. Subsequently his verbal output decreased, and he only engaged in short conversations. Prior blood and CSF laboratory evaluations ruled out causes of rapidly progressive dementia (see Case 34). A trial of rivastigmine 3 mg twice daily provided no clear benefit. By the time of his evaluation, he needed assistance with all activities of daily living, could not ambulate independently, and swallowing was impaired. His exam showed a symmetric parkinsonism with retrocollis. On oculomotor exam, range of vertical motion was limited (Video 8.1). However, his spouse commented this was unusual for him. The rest of the exam was limited due to his inability to follow commands. He had not been exposed to antipsychotics or antiemetic medications in the past. Given the presence of retrocollis, mild appendicular, marked axial rigidity, and ophthalmoplegia, he was given the diagnosis of rapidly deteriorating progressive supranuclear palsy (PSP). He returned to the clinic five years later, exhibiting progression to akinetic mutism (Video 8.2). His family reported he had been admitted multiple times for aspiration pneumonia. In addition, they reported that the addition of donepezil 10 mg daily had eliminated the hallucinations. He died seven months later. His autopsy demonstrated extensive Lewy bodies, particularly affecting cortical regions, meeting pathological criteria for diffuse Lewy body disease (DLBD).

Could This Have Been Recognized Earlier?

The initial assessment was anchored on the more prominent motor features, including retrocollis and axial rigidity. These are more often associated with

PSP. However, the presence of hallucinations and cognitive fluctuations are more often associated with underlying synucleinopathies rather than tauopathies (see Case 23) (Bertram and Williams, 2012; Williams et al., 2008). This should have raised the concern for DLB early in the course.

How about the Ophthalmoplegia?

In the context of parkinsonism and cognitive impairment, oculomotor abnormalities are highly suggestive of PSP. However, when the patient is unable to follow commands due to impaired alertness or attention, the validity of abnormal performance as a diagnostic sign is affected. This principle also applies to the evaluation of other cognitive and motor domains. In this case, the spouse mentioned he was having one of his "typical episodes of confusion," which should have been interpreted as a manifestation of the cognitive fluctuations she had previously described. The proper interpretation of this information would have deemphasized the findings of the oculomotor exam (also, the video demonstrates that the vertical range is not improved with the oculocephalic maneuver) and prioritized the presence of cognitive fluctuation in the assessment.

Discussion

The recognition of changes in arousal or vigilance is a challenging yet crucial aspect of the evaluation of cognitive impairment. Arousal, described as the general state of responsivity and wakefulness, represents the fundamental requirement for consciousness which enables all other cognitive operations. Attention can be defined as the preferential allocation of cognitive resources to events that have temporarily become relevant (Mesulam, 2010). This can be further subdivided into three subtypes: sustained, selective, and divided attention. Sustained attention or vigilance refers to the capacity of maintaining attentional activity over a prolonged period of time. The ability to focus on one stimulus while suppressing awareness of competing stimuli is known as selective attention, whereas divided attention describes the ability to respond to more than one task at once. Both selective and divided attention overlap significantly with executive function.

Video 8.1 The examination demonstrates marked retrocollis and hypomimia. When asked to move his eyes, he is unable to follow commands. He is mumbling something unintelligible during the exam. Note that at the end of the video, his spouse notices that this is unusual for him.

Video 8.2 Evaluation done five years later shows similar findings. Note again that the caregiver mentions that his ability to perform activities fluctuates.

The standard assessment of the cognitive domains assumes that the subject evaluated is fully awake and has normal vigilance. Cognitive testing results become unreliable in the context of impaired arousal or vigilance, as performance deficits may not reflect domain-specific impairments (Escandon et al., 2010). In clinic, impairments may be suspected during the interview when the patient appears drowsy or when questions need to be repeated multiple times. In the appropriate context, deficits in simple attention tests like forward digit span, cancellation tasks, or Trails A raise the concern for impaired arousal or vigilance.

Cognitive fluctuations are a common feature of DLB and are often reported as daytime drowsiness, excessive daytime naps, prolonged staring into space (i.e., being "out of it"), or disorganized speech. These fluctuations appear abruptly, interrupting an ongoing activity. The periodicity, duration, and severity of fluctuations are variable, even within the same patient (McKeith et al., 1996). Different from seizures, there are not motor or sensory changes, and carers may be able to interrupt these episodes by calling out the patient (Matar et al., 2019). The presence of fluctuations, particularly early in the disease, can be helpful to differentiate DLB from other neurodegenerative disorders, including Alzheimer disease (Ferman et al., 2004). A potentially treatable mechanism may be underlying dysautonomia, with episodes of hypotension or orthostatic hypotension explaining periods of transient cognitive worsening (Riley and Espay, 2018). However, cognitive fluctuations should not be confused with the minor day to day or diurnal/nocturnal variations (sundowning) that commonly occur in most patients with dementia of any etiology or unmasking of cognitive impairment by increased cognitive demand. Asking a question like "Are there episodes when his/her thinking seems quite clear and then becomes muddled?" is not helpful in determining the presence of fluctuations, as up to 75 percent of carers of patients with AD and DLB answer positively (Bradshaw et al., 2004). Multiple questionnaires and diaries with the purpose of characterizing

Table 8.1 Causes of fluctuations in arousal or vigilance

Category	Examples
Drugs	Anticholinergic burden (e.g., oxybutynin) Sedative burden (e.g., benzodiazepines, opioids, antihistamines) Drugs of abuse (e.g., ethanol, opiates) Withdrawal states (e.g., ethanol, benzodiazepines)
Infections	Sepsis Encephalitis/meningitis Urinary tract infection
Metabolic abnormalities	Electrolyte disturbance (e.g., hyponatremia, hypercalcemia) Endocrine abnormalities (e.g., hypothyroidism, adrenal insufficiency) Hyperglycemia and hypoglycemia
System organ failure	Cardiac failure Renal failure Liver failure Pulmonary disease
Other	Hypertension or hypotension Epileptic seizures Sleep apnea

the characteristics of fluctuations have been developed. These include the Clinician Assessment of Fluctuation (CAF), One Day Fluctuation Assessment Scale, and Mayo Fluctuations Composite Scale (Ferman et al., 2004; Walker et al., 2000). Finally, impaired arousal or vigilance is also a feature of delirium that should be ruled out as part of initial diagnostic evaluation. In addition, other processes can lead or contribute to fluctuations in arousal or vigilance, without necessarily causing delirium (Table 8.1).

Diagnosis: Dementia with Lewy bodies

Tip: Hallucinations and cognitive fluctuations suggest an underlying synucleinopathy. Impairments of arousal or attention during the exam affect the interpretation of the findings.

References

Bertram, K. and Williams, D. R. 2012. Visual hallucinations in the differential diagnosis of parkinsonism. *J Neurol Neurosurg Psychiatry* **83**(4) 448–452.

Bradshaw, J. et al. 2004. Fluctuating cognition in dementia with Lewy bodies and Alzheimer's disease is qualitatively distinct. *J Neurol Neurosurg Psychiatry* **75**(3) 382–387.

Escandon, A., Al-Hammadi, N. and Galvin, J. E. 2010. Effect of cognitive fluctuation on neuropsychological performance in aging and dementia. *Neurology* **74**(3) 210–217.

Ferman, T. J. et al. 2004. DLB fluctuations: specific features that reliably differentiate DLB from AD and normal aging. *Neurology* **62**(2) 181–187.

Matar, E., Shine, J. M., Halliday, G. M. and Lewis, S. J. G. 2019. Cognitive fluctuations in Lewy body dementia: towards a pathophysiological framework. *Brain* 1 31–46.

McKeith, I. G. et al. 1996. Consensus guidelines for the clinical and pathologic diagnosis of dementia with Lewy bodies (DLB). *Neurology* **47**(5) 1113.

Mesulam, M. M. 2010. Attentional and confusional States. *Continuum* **16**(4) 128–139.

Riley, D. E. and Espay, A. J. 2018. Cognitive fluctuations in Parkinson's disease dementia: blood pressure lability as an underlying mechanism. *J Clin Mov Disord* **5** 1.

Walker, M. P. et al. 2000. The clinician assessment of fluctuation and the one day fluctuation assessment scale: two methods to assess fluctuating confusion in dementia. *Br J Psychiatry* **177** 252–256.

Williams, D. R., Warren, J. D. and Lees, A. J. 2008. Using the presence of visual hallucinations to differentiate Parkinson's disease from atypical parkinsonism. *J Neurol Neurosurg Psychiatry* **79**(6) 652–655.

Case: This 61-year-old right-handed woman presented with a 5-year history of progressive cognitive, behavioral, and gait impairment. She was first noticed to be withdrawn, exhibiting a decreased level of energy and interest, after her father's death seven years earlier. Previously abstemious to alcohol and strict on her diet because of diabetes, she started drinking a bottle of wine per day and eating more sweets. These were thought to be coping mechanisms to deal with depression. Her behavior continued to decline despite antidepressant treatment with citalopram 40 mg, which she had been on for four years. Most of the day, she would watch TV, no longer engaging in her prior hobbies (gardening and knitting). She became more impolite and irritable, also distractible and disorganized, requiring prompts and detailed instructions for simple tasks. Her credit card was cancelled due to inability to manage her finances and excessive shopping. Her husband noticed that she was more distant and no longer expressed interest in her family members. Attributing these changes to depression and alcohol intake, her family restricted her access to alcohol, and she abruptly stopped drinking. By the time of her assessment, there had been no alcohol intake for two years. However, her condition continued to deteriorate. Over the previous year, she reported balance impairment but no falls. There was neither personal premorbid psychiatric history nor family history of neurological or psychiatric disease.

On examination, she exhibited a flat affect and was easily distracted. She endorsed balance problems but denied any cognitive or behavioral problems. Although she denied feeling sad, she acknowledged that she was no longer interested in her hobbies. Exam revealed bradykinesia and her gait was wide based with absent arm swing. Montreal Cognitive Assessment (MoCA) score was 21/30 due to impairments in trail making, cube copy and clock drawing, forward and backward digit span, phonemic fluency, and delayed recall (she recalled three words freely and recognized the other two when multiple choices were given).

Should We Attribute Her Presentation to Suboptimal Management of Depression?

Despite meeting criteria for depression, multiple elements of her presentation argue against the diagnosis. First, lack of interest and initiative in the absence of sadness, worthlessness, or guilt suggested apathy rather than depression. Second, the presence of personality changes (e.g., impoliteness and lack of empathy) in addition to the development of new habits (e.g., alcohol consumption and impulsive shopping) is not typically associated with depression. Moreover, the severity of the dysexecutive pattern of cognitive impairment is beyond what can be accounted for in depression (see Case 2). Finally, the parkinsonian features with progressive gait impairment for two years suggested a neurodegenerative disorder.

Her progressive behavioral and cognitive changes were consistent with the behavioral variant of frontotemporal dementia (bvFTD). Although parkinsonism is not embedded into the diagnostic criteria, it is frequently seen as the condition progresses. The brain MRI showed a pattern of regional atrophy predominantly affecting the frontal lobes (Figure 9.1), supporting the clinical diagnosis of probable bvFTD.

Discussion

Apathy is a syndrome characterized by decreased motivation manifesting as a change in responsiveness to internal and external stimuli (Robert et al., 2009). As a syndrome, apathy encompasses behavioral, cognitive, and affective domains (Table 9.1) (Robert et al., 2009). Apathy is common in patients with neurodegenerative disorders, stroke, and brain injury (Lanctôt et al., 2017). In neurodegenerative disorders, apathy is frequently present at the onset, where it may be misdiagnosed as depression. The presence of apathy has a significant adverse impact on a patient's safety, independence, and quality of life, in addition to increasing the burden of care (Chow et al., 2009).

Patients typically have poor insight regarding these symptoms, while caregivers may perceive it as depression or to mobility restrictions. Although apathy and depression may coexist, distinguishing them is key to guide treatment (Table 9.2). In the

Table 9.1 Subdomains of apathy: Clinical features and potential treatments

Domain	Behavioral	Cognitive	Affective
Clinical features	Impaired self-initiated behavior • Starting conversation • Doing basic daily activities Impaired response to environment-stimulated behavior • Responding to conversation • Participating in social activities	Cognitive inertia • Lack of spontaneous ideas • Lack of interest in new stimuli • Lack of curiosity	Impaired spontaneous emotion • Blunted affect • Report of absence of emotions Loss of emotional responsiveness to external stimuli • Lack of emotion to relevant personal events
Medications to consider	Dopamine receptor agonists[a] • Pramipexole • Ropinirole • Rotigotine • Piribedil	Acetylcholinesterase Inhibitors[b] • Donepezil • Rivastigmine • Galantamine	Dopamine receptor agonists[a] • Pramipexole • Ropinirole • Rotigotine • Piribedil Methylphenidate Amphetamine Bupropion

[a] Dopamine agonists should be used with caution, particularly in frontotemporal dementia, Parkinson disease with and without dementia, and dementia with Lewy bodies, as they may cause impulse control disorders and psychosis.
[b] Acetylcholinesterase inhibitors are not recommended for patients with frontotemporal dementia.

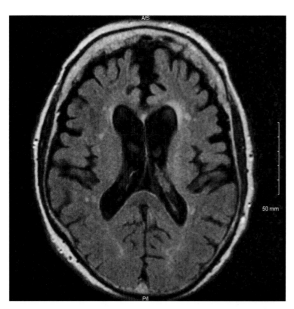

Figure 9.1 FLAIR axial brain MRI in this patient. Note the frontal lobe atrophy.

context of decreased motivation, the absence of sadness (i.e., lack of mood disturbance), hopelessness, guilt, or suicidality (i.e., lack of cognitive symptoms of depression) should raise the suspicion for apathy rather than depression (Stanton and Carson, 2016). Pharmacotherapy is different for those with depression without apathy, apathy without depression, and those with both ("apathetic depression"). Activating antidepressants, such as serotonin–norepinephrine reuptake inhibitors (SNRIs), may be considered as the first choice for apathy, while selective serotonin reuptake inhibitors (SSRIs) may actually worsen apathy symptoms (Wongpakaran et al., 2007). If the trial is ineffective after at least two months at a dose within the therapeutic range, the medication should be discontinued. Apathy subdomain identification (i.e., behavioral, cognitive, or affective) can guide treatment approach, although the evidence for this approach is based on case reports and case series (Table 9.1) (Marin et al., 1995). In addition, nonpharmacological measures, including establishing routines and using prompts, are recommended.

Diagnosis: Behavioral variant of frontotemporal dementia (bvFTD) presenting with apathy

Tip: Lack of interest and initiative in the absence of sadness and cognitive symptoms of depression should raise concerns for apathy rather than depression. Identifying the manifestations of the different domains of apathy helps guide management.

Table 9.2 Distinctive and shared features of depression and apathy and potential treatments.

Depression	Apathy	Both
• Sadness • Feelings of guilt • Hopelessness • Pessimism • Self-criticism • Diurnal variation in mood • Anxiety • Suicidal ideation	• Reduced initiative • Lack of spontaneous interest in participating in activities • Emotional indifference • Diminished emotional reactivity • Lack of concern for others	• Psychomotor slowing • Anhedonia • Lack of energy • Decreased interest/ engagement in usual pursuits
Treatments to consider		

• SSRIs
  o Sertraline
  o Citalopram
• SNRIs
  o Venlafaxine
  o Duloxetine
• Bupropion
	• Dopamine agonists[a]
	  o Pramipexole
	  o Ropinirole
	  o Rotigotine
	  o Piribedil
	• Acetylcholinesterase inhibitors[b]
	  o Donepezil
	  o Rivastigmine
	  o Galantamine
	• Methylphenidate
	• Amphetamine
	• Bupropion
		• SNRIs
		  o Venlafaxine
		• Combination therapies (as above, except SSRIs)

Note: SNRIs: serotonin–norepinephrine reuptake inhibitor; SSRIs: selective serotonin reuptake inhibitor.

[a] Dopamine agonists should be used with caution particularly in frontotemporal dementia, Parkinson disease with and without dementia, and dementia with Lewy bodies as they may cause impulse control disorders.

[b] Acetylcholinesterase inhibitors are not recommended in frontotemporal dementia.

References

Chow, T. W. et al. 2009. Apathy symptom profile and behavioral associations in frontotemporal dementia vs dementia of Alzheimer type. *Arch Neurol* **66**(7) 888–893.

Lanctôt, K. L. et al. 2017. Apathy associated with neurocognitive disorders: recent progress and future directions. *Alzheimers Dement* **13**(1) 84–100.

Marin, R. S. et al. 1995. Apathy: a treatable syndrome. *J Neuropsychiatry Clin Neurosci* **7**(1) 23–30.

Robert, P. et al. 2009. Proposed diagnostic criteria for apathy in Alzheimer's disease and other neuropsychiatric disorders. *Eur Psychiatry* **24**(2) 98–104.

Stanton, B. R. and Carson, A. 2016. Apathy: a practical guide for neurologists. *Pract Neurol* **16**(1) 42–47.

Wongpakaran, N., van Reekum, R., Wongpakaran, T. and Clarke, D. 2007. Selective serotonin reuptake inhibitor use associates with apathy among depressed elderly: a case-control study. *Ann Gen Psychiatry* **6** 7.

Case: This 56-year-old right-handed man presented with a 3-year history of progressive difficulties with vision. He first noticed problems reading on the computer, which he attributed to misrecognizing letters and words. In addition, he had trouble finding objects once he had put them down, particularly if placed among others. His family noticed dressing appeared to be more challenging for him, though he felt this was a minor issue. He denied any difficulty recognizing object or faces. Neither he nor his family felt there were memory problems. While he endorsed some subtle problems with word finding, he acknowledged his language was otherwise normal. He felt that his mood was reasonably good, and his family agreed. He had to move in with his son as he gave up driving because of visual difficulties.

His exam was remarkable for optic ataxia (impairment reaching a target under visual guidance), oculomotor apraxia (a deficit initiating voluntary eye movements), and simultanagnosia (missing the whole of a visual scene for its parts). There was no evidence of limb apraxia. Montreal Cognitive Assessment (MoCA) score was 19/30 due to impairments in trail making, cube copying, clock drawing, backward digit span, serial sevens, and delayed recall (he recalled three words freely, and recognized the other two when multiple choices were given).

Should He Be Referred to an Ophthalmologist?

While most of the changes are related to vision, they do not imply ocular pathology. On the contrary, the presence of simultanagnosia, optic ataxia, and oculomotor apraxia suggest Balint syndrome, which is associated with bilateral parieto-occipital disruption. In addition, he presents with acalculia and dressing apraxia, which also suggest parietal pathology.

Formal neuropsychological testing revealed visual-spatial and perceptual deficits. On the Visual Object Spatial Perceptual Battery, he was unable to see any of 10 fragmented letters and could not count any of the 3D cubes. He recognized 9/10 famous faces that were presented to him. He scored 19/30 on the Sydney Language Battery confrontational naming test, which is suggestive of anomia. He had preserved color naming and color matching. In comparison, he performed at average on the auditory verbal learning test (AVLT) of memory.

His MRI scan showed biparietal atrophy while his FDG-PET scan revealed biparietal and occipital hypometabolism, which was slightly worse on the right (Figure 10.1). His clinical presentation and posterior hypometabolism were consistent with posterior cortical atrophy. The amyloid PET scan was visually read as positive with a moderate amount of beta-amyloid deposition, indicative of Alzheimer disease.

Discussion

Posterior cortical atrophy (PCA) is a syndrome associated with neurodegeneration of the occipital and parietal lobes primarily (Crutch et al., 2017). Alzheimer disease (AD) is the pathology most often associated with PCA, followed by dementia with Lewy bodies (DLB) (often in combination with AD pathology), corticobasal degeneration, and prion disease (Renner et al., 2004). Diagnostic criteria rely on the presence of clinical and imaging findings localized to bilateral occipital and parietal lobes (Table 10.1) (Crutch et al., 2017).

Visuospatial and perceptual deficits encompass a number of impairments associated with the involvement of the primary visual cortex and the visual processing streams (see Case 29). Hallucinations should raise the concern for a DLB diagnosis (Josephs et al., 2006). In addition, features of the Gerstmann syndrome, a combination acalculia, left-right disorientation, finger agnosia, and agraphia, may be observed when the dominant angular gyrus is affected (Rusconi, 2018). However, agraphia is not included as a criteria for PCA. Finally, apraxia, often manifesting as difficulties performing learned complex movements, including dressing, reflects dominant parietal degeneration. Memory, executive function, and language are preserved early in the disease (McMonagle et al., 2006). There can be pseudo-anomia in the setting of impairment of visual processing, whereby the inability to translate the visual information about the object manifests as an inability to name it. Subjects usually have insight into their deficits, and their behavior and personality are not affected early in the disease (Schott and Crutch, 2019).

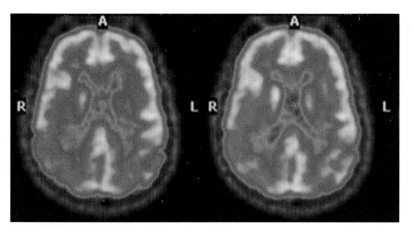

Figure 10.1 FDG-PET in this patient. Note the biparietal and occipital hypometabolism, which is slightly worse on the right. For the colour version, please refer to the plate section.

Except for subtle myoclonus, the remainder of the neurological examination is often unremarkable in PCA due to AD. Parkinsonism in the context of hallucinations, anosmia, or dream enactment behavior suggests DLB instead (Ryan et al., 2014). Markedly asymmetric motor findings, including myoclonus, dystonia, and alien limb, suggest corticobasal degeneration (Ryan et al., 2014). Rapid progression of symptoms should raise the concern for prion disease, particularly the Heidenhain variant of Creutzfeldt–Jakob disease, which may include frightening visual distortions (Crutch et al., 2017).

Structural imaging demonstrates an atrophy pattern predominantly affecting the occipital and parietal lobes, often sparing the hippocampi. Fluorodeoxyglucose positron emission tomography (FDG-PET) reveals hypometabolism within the parieto-occipital cortices (Nestor et al., 2003). Amyloid imaging is helpful to determine if AD is the underlying pathology. While PCA reflects a focal neurodegenerative process, the presence of amyloid is usually diffused in AD cases, limiting its ability to distinguish between AD syndromes (Rosenbloom et al., 2011). This differs from tau imaging where a more significant signal is seen in the areas correlating with the clinical presentation (Ossenkoppele et al., 2015). AD cerebrospinal fluid biomarkers are helpful to determine underlying AD. However, it should be noted that levels of total and phosphorylated tau are not as high in PCA when compared to typical AD. This difference is attributed to the extent of neurodegeneration (Paterson et al., 2015).

Management remains symptomatic and varies according to the underlying pathology. Cholinesterase inhibitors and memantine are appropriate when AD or DLB is suspected. As patients usually have insight into their deficits and the limitations, depression and anxiety need to be assessed and treated appropriately. Besides medications, explaining the nature of the condition and what to expect is of paramount importance for patients and caregivers. The need to adapt to the patient's present and future limitations with safety as a priority should be stressed (Table 10.2). While most patients are no longer driving by the time of the diagnosis, the abilities of those who are should be comprehensively and frequently evaluated.

Diagnosis: Posterior cortical atrophy due to Alzheimer disease

Tip: Progressive visuospatial deficits and agnosia along with apraxia and Gertsmann syndrome should raise the concern for posterior cortical atrophy. Alzheimer disease is the most likely etiology. However, the presence of parkinsonism and markedly asymmetric findings should raise the concern for underlying dementia with Lewy bodies and corticobasal syndrome, respectively.

References

Crutch, S. J. et al. 2017. Consensus classification of posterior cortical atrophy. *Alzheimers Dement* **13**(8) 870–884.

Josephs, K. A. et al. 2006. Visual hallucinations in posterior cortical atrophy. *Arch Neurol* **63**(10) 1427–1432.

McMonagle, P., Deering, F., Berliner, Y. and Kertesz, A. 2006. The cognitive profile of posterior cortical atrophy. *Neurology* **66**(3) 331–338.

Nestor, P. J. et al. 2003. The topography of metabolic deficits in posterior cortical atrophy (the visual variant of Alzheimer's disease) with FDG-PET. *J Neurol Neurosurg Psychiatry* **74**(11) 1521–1529.

Table 10.1 Core features of the posterior cortical atrophy syndrome

Clinical features

- Insidious onset
- Gradual progression
- Prominent early disturbance of visual with or without other posterior cognitive functions

Cognitive features (at least any three in any category need to be present early in the course of the disease)

- Temporo-occipital
  - o Object perception deficit
  - o Environmental agnosia
  - o Apperceptive prosopagnosia
  - o Alexia
  - o Homonymous visual field defect

- Parietal
  - o Spatial perception deficit
  - o Constructional dyspraxia
  - o Limb apraxia
  - o Dressing apraxia
  - o Balint syndrome[a]
    - Simultanagnosia
    - Oculomotor apraxia
    - Optic ataxia
  - o Gerstmann syndrome[a]
    - Left/right disorientation
    - Acalculia
    - Finger agnosia

Relatively spared
- Anterograde memory function
- Speech and nonvisual language function
- Executive function
- Behavior and personality

Neuroimaging

- Evidence of occipitotemporal or occipitoparietal degeneration
  - o Atrophy in MRI
  - o Hypometabolism in FDG-PET
  - o Hypoperfusion in SPECT

Exclusion criteria
- Evidence of a brain tumor or other mass lesion sufficient to explain the symptom
- Evidence of significant vascular disease including focal stroke sufficient to explain the symptoms
- Evidence of afferent visual cause (e.g., optic nerve, chiasm, or tract)
- Evidence of other identifiable causes for cognitive impairment (e.g., renal failure)

Note: FDG-PET: 18F-labeled fluorodeoxyglucose positron emission tomography; MRI: magnetic resonance imaging; SPECT: single-photon emission computed tomography.

[a] Each component within the syndrome is counted independently. Agraphia is part of Gerstmann syndrome but not included in the criteria for PCA.

Source: Adapted from Crutch et al. (2017).

Table 10.2 Selected suggestions on home adaptions for patients with posterior cortical atrophy

Simplify the environment

- Ensure adequate lighting, particularly at nightfall.
- Remove clutter and objects no longer in use; keep pathways clear.
- Remove unsafe furniture (e.g., low-height stools), rugs, and mats.
- Cover mirrors if necessary: often people with vision problems may not be able to recognize the item as a mirror.
- Place cleaning supplies away from food supplies.
- Set up a "memory center" with the phone, keys, note pad, whiteboard with large writing area, and black marker.

Make objects easy to identify

- Label room doors, drawers, and shelves using yellow paper with black writing.
- Paint doorframes and light switch plates in a contrasting color to the wall.
- Use contrasting-colored adhesive strips to mark pathways to important areas – bathroom, kitchen, living room, laundry.
- Use solid colors for objects that contrast with the background (e.g., dark plates on light table mat).

Maintain a structure

- Maintain a strict pattern for setup of elements of use (e.g., utensils during meals or bathroom items).

Security additions

- Railing and safety gate on stairs
- Contrasting-colored tape or paint on the edge of each step
- Nonslip bathmat and high-contrast grab bars in the shower
- Phone with large print and high-contrast numbers, as well as one-touch programmable numbers
- Programed emergency and frequently used numbers to the one-touch phone and added tactile markers to increase ease of identification

Source: Adapted from Schott and Crutch (2019).

Ossenkoppele, R. et al. 2015. Tau, amyloid, and hypometabolism in a patient with posterior cortical atrophy. *Ann Neurol* **77**(2) 338–342.

Paterson, R. W. et al. 2015. Dissecting IWG-2 typical and atypical Alzheimer's disease: insights from cerebrospinal fluid analysis. *J Neurol* **262**(12) 2722–2730.

Renner, J. A. et al. 2004. Progressive posterior cortical dysfunction: a clinicopathologic series. *Neurology* **63**(7) 1175–1180.

Rosenbloom, M. H. et al. 2011. Distinct clinical and metabolic deficits in PCA and AD are not related to amyloid distribution. *Neurology* **76**(21) 1789–1796.

Rusconi, E. 2018. Gerstmann syndrome: historic and current perspectives. *Handb Clin Neurol* **151** 395–411.

Ryan, N. S. et al. 2014. Motor features in posterior cortical atrophy and their imaging correlates. *Neurobiol Aging* **35**(12) 2845–2857.

Schott, J. M. and Crutch, S. J. 2019. Posterior cortical atrophy. *Continuum* **25**(1) 52–75.

CASE 11 | The Stroke of Clarity

Case: This 75-year-old right-handed woman presented with a nine-month history of progressive cognitive impairment. Her children reported that the first problem was, abruptly, an inability for her to see things on the left side of her visual field. In the hospital, she was found to have left homonymous hemianopia associated with a stroke in the right occipital lobe. During her admission she appeared disoriented, claiming she was at her mother's house. Repeat imaging was unchanged, and metabolic and infectious workups did not show abnormalities. She returned to baseline before the discharge. After her discharge, her children noted progressive decline. She became increasingly forgetful about recent events and repetitive in her questions and statements. Due to the temporal correlation between these symptoms and the stroke, she was diagnosed with poststroke dementia.

On exam, nine months after the first deficit, she was alert, oriented to person and place. She was able to only follow one-step commands. Her speech was fluent, but her discourse was circumlocutory. Other than subtle left inferior quadrantanopsia, the remainder of her examination was unremarkable. Cognitive evaluation revealed impaired encoding: she was able to recall 3 words out of 10 after three trials and recognized only the same 3 after. She showed deficits in naming and verbal fluency, semantic was worse than phonemic. Her visuospatial abilities were within normal limits. A repeat brain MRI was reported as unchanged with no

thalamic involvement (which can be involved in posterior cerebral artery strokes). Careful review also showed mild generalized atrophy, with hippocampal involvement (Figure 11.1).

Does the Stroke Localization Help Explain the Pattern of Cognitive Changes?

Strokes affecting the occipital lobe are frequently associated with primary visual deficits rather than cognitive or behavioral deficits. The stroke caused her quadrantopsia. However, her progressive amnestic cognitive deficits in the context of hippocampal atrophy in absence of further infarcts suggests a neurodegenerative process, most likely Alzheimer disease.

How Would You Explain the Abrupt Onset of Symptoms in the Context of an Acute Stroke?

The possibility of gradual change in cognition that became evident after an unrelated acute event must always be considered. It is not uncommon for families to report an abrupt or rapid cognitive decline in patients with slowly progressive neurodegenerative conditions. Unrelated disorders (e.g., infection, metabolic abnormality) can lower the threshold for the

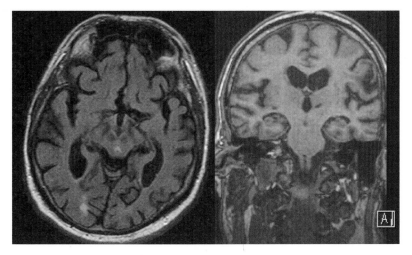

Figure 11.1 FLAIR axial and coronal brain MRI in this patient. Note the poststroke gliosis affecting the right occipital lobe as well as the diffuse cortical atrophy on the axial image and the bilateral hippocampal atrophy on the coronal section.

Table 11.1 Short form of the Informant Questionnaire on Cognitive Decline in the Elderly
"Now we want you to remember what your friend or relative was like 10 years ago and to compare it with what he/she is like now. 10 years ago was in 20___."* Below are situations where this person has to use his/her memory or intelligence and we want you to indicate whether this has improved, stayed the same or got worse in that situation over the past 10 years. Note the importance of comparing his/her present performance with 10 years ago. So if 10 years ago this person always forgot where he/she had left things, and he/she still does, then this would be considered "Hasn't changed much." Please indicate the changes you have observed by circling the appropriate answer. Compared with 10 years ago how is this person at:

	1	2	3	4	5
Remembering things about family and friends, e.g., occupations, birthdays, addresses?	Much improved	A bit improved	Not much changed	A bit worse	Much worse
Remembering things that have happened recently?	Much improved	A bit improved	Not much changed	A bit worse	Much worse
Recalling conversations a few days later?	Much improved	A bit improved	Not much changed	A bit worse	Much worse
Remembering his/her address and telephone number?	Much improved	A bit improved	Not much changed	A bit worse	Much worse
Remembering what day and month it is?	Much improved	A bit improved	Not much changed	A bit worse	Much worse
Remembering where things are usually kept?	Much improved	A bit improved	Not much changed	A bit worse	Much worse
Remembering where to find things that have been put in a different place from usual?	Much improved	A bit improved	Not much changed	A bit worse	Much worse
Knowing how to work familiar machines around the house?	Much improved	A bit improved	Not much changed	A bit worse	Much worse
Learning to use a new gadget or machine around the house?	Much improved	A bit improved	Not much changed	A bit worse	Much worse
Learning new things in general?	Much improved	A bit improved	Not much changed	A bit worse	Much worse
Following a story in a book or on TV?	Much improved	A bit improved	Not much changed	A bit worse	Much worse
Making decisions on everyday matters?	Much improved	A bit improved	Not much changed	A bit worse	Much worse
Handling money for shopping?	Much improved	A bit improved	Not much changed	A bit worse	Much worse
Handling financial matters?	Much improved	A bit improved	Not much changed	A bit worse	Much worse
Handling other everyday arithmetic problems?	Much improved	A bit improved	Not much changed	A bit worse	Much worse
Using his/her intelligence to understand what is going on and to reason things through?	Much improved	A bit improved	Not much changed	A bit worse	Much worse

Note: Short IQCODE, by A. F. Jorm (1994).

manifestations of neurodegenerative disorders to become evident. However, some factors need to be considered when assuming normal cognition before a certain event or period. The first is the premorbid level of activity and routine. Subjects with cognitive impairment tend to favor a restricted routine which is less challenging and frustrating than the pursuit of novel activities. Difficulties adapting to new environments (e.g., social events or a new home) or tasks (e.g., using a new cell phone) may be the first sign of

Table 11.2 Selected cognitive and behavioral deficits associated with isolated strokes of subcortical structures

Stroke localization	Cognitive/behavioral deficits
Thalamus – anterior	Amnesia, abulia, neglect, nonfluent aphasia
Thalamus – paramedian	Altered level of alertness, amnesia, abulia, confabulations
Thalamus – posterior	Fluent aphasia and neglect
Caudate	Dysexecutive syndrome, impaired sustained attention, apathy, agitation
Putamen	Aphasia, neglect, apathy
Globus pallidus	Abulia
Inferior genu of the internal capsule	Altered level of alertness, abulia, dysexecutive syndrome

cognitive impairment. The second factor is the insight family and caregivers have at different stages about a patient's function. In this case, the stroke focused the patient's children on her daily activities and thus they became more aware of her cognitive changes.

In this case, although her children were not aware of subtle changes before the stroke, they became aware her cognitive changes were progressive, and were affecting basic activities. Most likely, her cognitive impairment had been overlooked for years before the stroke. Her social isolation and simple routine disguised her cognitive impairment. Her admission to the hospital, precipitated by a stroke, lead to closer observation which made her family aware of changes that could not have been attributed to the stroke.

Discussion

Cognitive deficits are commonly seen after acute strokes (Godefroy and Bogousslavsky, 2007). However, determining if the extent of cerebrovascular injury suffices to account for the cognitive deficits remains a significant challenge (Smith, 2016).

The emergence of cognitive of deficits after a stroke is a compelling argument to associate both. However, overlooking a history of cognitive decline preceding the stroke is a common pitfall, leading to misdiagnosis. In order to avoid delaying the recognition of a neurodegenerative process, thorough questioning of the subject's baseline cognitive abilities should always be emphasized. Was functioning truly normal, even if a "magnifying glass" were to have been used before the acute event? Was she doing everything she had always done or, instead, restricting her routine? Formal questionnaires like the Informant Questionnaire on Cognitive Decline in the Elderly (IQCODE) can be helpful in these situations (Jorm, 1994). The short form is available without copyright protection (Table 11.1) (Jorm, 1994).

The number, volume, and location of strokes can affect the risk of poststroke cognitive impairment. Single strategic locations have been associated with certain cognitive deficits. These are more clearly established for strokes affecting cortical structures (Godefroy and Bogousslavsky, 2007). However, strategic strokes in subcortical structures may present with a number of cognitive and behavioral deficits (Table 11.2) (Ferro, 2001; Godefroy and Bogousslavsky, 2007; Mori, 2002). Although these deficits tend to improve or remain stable after the stroke, fluctuations in alertness and cognition have been described in the context of thalamic strokes (Schmahmann, 2003). In addition, thalamic infarcts may present with memory impairment, affecting not only encoding but also retrieval (i.e., anterograde and retrograde amnesia). Some cases may be associated with confabulation due to the involvement of the mamilothalamic tract (Schmahmann, 2003).

Diagnosis: Alzheimer disease made apparent after an unrelated acute event

Tip: Cognitive impairment is unlikely after brain lesions affecting a region not associated with cognitive deficits. After an acute event, recognizing deficits as progressive and carefully defining the subject's prior cognitive abilities, scope of his/her activities over time, and level of caregiver's insight are critical to establishing the appropriate diagnosis.

References

Ferro, J. M. 2001. Hyperacute cognitive stroke syndromes. *J Neurol* **248**(10) 841–849.

Godefroy, O. and Bogousslavsky, J. 2007. *The Behavioral and Cognitive Neurology of Stroke*. Cambridge, UK: Cambridge University Press.

Jorm, A. F. 1994. A short form of the Informant Questionnaire on Cognitive Decline in the Elderly (IQCODE): development and cross-validation. *Psychol Med* **24**(1) 145–153.

Mori, E. 2002. Impact of subcortical ischemic lesions on behavior and cognition. *Ann N Y Acad Sci* **977** 141–148.

Schmahmann, J. D. 2003. Vascular syndromes of the thalamus. *Stroke* **34**(9) 2264–2278.

Smith, E. 2016. Vascular cognitive impairment. *Continuum* **22**(2) 490–509.

Case: This 57-year-old right-handed woman presented to the clinic after four episodes of amnesia. The first one occurred six months previously while at her daughter's house. Abruptly, she became disoriented to location and situation. She knew who she was and could recognize her daughter. She was reoriented by her daughter multiple times but still repeatedly asked where she was. She was taken to the emergency room, and after 45 minutes, she returned to her baseline and could recall the episode of disorientation. Her neurological exam was unremarkable, as well as her laboratory investigations, brain MRI, and EEG. She was discharged back home with the diagnosis of transient global amnesia (TGA). She had three additional episodes of similar characteristics since then, all within the last two months. She was on treatment with amlodipine for hypertension. Her repeat exam in the office setting was unremarkable.

Are These Features Fully Consistent with Transient Global Amnesia?

Recurrence of TGA is uncommon, particularly episodes within months of each other. This alone raises the concern for an alternative diagnosis. In addition, the duration of the episodes reported here were shorter than what is usually observed in TGA. Finally, her ability to recall the episode represents another red flag in the diagnosis of TGA, where patients usually describe a gap in their memory. These features suggest transient epileptic amnesia (TEA) rather than TGA (Butler et al., 2007). Further inquiry must include the presence of aura (e.g., olfactory hallucinosis), automatisms (e.g., lip smacking or chewing), and whether the episodes occur on waking, all of which are suggestive of an epileptic cause. Brain MRI and EEG should be repeated. The EEG should be preferably done while sleep deprived to increase the likelihood of finding an abnormality.

Brain structural MRI was unremarkable. Sleep-deprived EEG showed temporal spikes, suggestive of epileptic activity. She was started on lamotrigine, and the dose was gradually increased to 125 mg twice a day. She has remained free of episodes after six months of follow-up.

Discussion

TGA represents the classic example of a transient amnesic syndrome, typically presenting between the ages of 50 and 70 years (Bartsch and Butler, 2013). Although the pathophysiology is not well defined, there is agreement regarding the involvement of the CA1 region of the hippocampus (Bartsch and Deuschl, 2010). The abrupt onset of impairment in memory encoding (i.e., forming new memories) is the key feature. Retrieval of autobiographical memories is usually impaired as well, with recent memories being more affected than older ones. Semantic and procedural memories are usually spared. Patients are aware of who they are but loose spatial and situational orientation, which is manifested with their multiple attempts to reorient themselves (e.g., asking multiple times "Where am I?" or "What am I doing here?"). Although patients may sense there is something wrong, but they are not aware of their deficits, which leads to significant anxiety and agitation. Headache, nausea, and dizziness may be present. Otherwise, no other cognitive or physical symptoms are present. The episode is self-limited (i.e., up to 24 hours), with most cases resolving in 4 to 8 hours. The recovery is complete without residual deficits. However, subjects are not able to recall what happened during the episode or the moments prior to it. Witnesses describe the episode being preceded by physical (e.g., diving into cold water) or emotional (e.g., receiving sad news) stressors. Recurrence is unusual, with up to 10 percent having a second or third event. Imaging during the event is typically unremarkable. However, focal punctuate DWI and T2-weighted lesions in the CA1 region of the hippocampus may be detected 2–4 days after the episode, disappearing after 14 days (Lee et al., 2007). EEG is typically normal.

The evaluation of an amnesic syndrome of abrupt onset, whether it is in the acute phase or after its resolution, requires the consideration of mimics of TGA. The two most common differential diagnoses are functional (i.e., dissociative amnesia in DSM-5) and transient epileptic amnesia (Table 12.1). In the former, retrograde memory is profoundly affected (sometimes selectively toward specific events), while the ability to form new memories is preserved, and patients also lose knowledge

Table 12.1 Main clinical features of selected transient amnesic syndromes

	Transient global amnesia	Transient epileptic amnesia	Dissociative amnesia
Anterograde memory	Impaired	Impaired	Normal or mildly impaired
Retrograde memory	Recent memories more impaired than distant ones	Recent memories more impaired than distant ones	Marked amnesia of a defined period of time
Other memory modalities (e.g., semantic, procedural)	Preserved	Preserved	May be impaired
Self-identity	Preserved	Preserved	Impaired
Duration	< 24 hours (usually 4–8 hours)	< 60 minutes	Minutes to days
Recurrence	Rare	Common	Variable

of their personal identity (they do not know who they are or do not recall such identifying information as their date of birth) (Markowitsch and Staniloiu, 2016). Deficits in procedural memory (e.g., how to use the cell phone) and the prolonged duration of events represent other useful clues (Markowitsch and Staniloiu, 2016). In the case of TEA (discussed earlier), patients may be initially diagnosed with Alzheimer disease based on their amnestic features. However, the episodic nature of the amnesia with normal functioning between episodes and lack of significant hippocampal atrophy favors TEA, instead. Other TGA mimics include strategic strokes affecting the hippocampi or anterior thalamus may present with additional deficits (e.g., aphasia, paresis) as well as evidence of ischemia on brain MRI (Giannantoni et al., 2015). Toxic-metabolic causes (e.g., sedatives, hypoglycemia) are frequently associated with an impaired level of alertness and attention (i.e., features of delirium), unlike TGA. Episodes of amnesia may also occur after head trauma and electroconvulsive therapy (ECT). Amnesia can be the presenting symptom of limbic encephalitis, although the onset tends to be subacute and is usually accompanied by other behavioral and cognitive changes, as well as evidence of involvement of the limbic system on MRI (Bartsch and Butler, 2013).

Diagnosis: Transient epileptic amnesia

Tip: Helpful variables to ascertain in the evaluation of a transient amnesic syndrome are the pattern of memory loss (e.g., anterograde, retrograde, semantic), the duration and any recurrences, and whether personal identity is compromised. Brain MRI and EEG are warranted in all patients.

References

Bartsch, T. and Butler, C. 2013. Transient amnesic syndromes. *Nat Rev Neurol* **9**(2) 86–97.

Bartsch, T. and Deuschl, G. 2010. Transient global amnesia: functional anatomy and clinical implications. *Lancet Neurol* **9**(2) 205–214.

Butler, C. R. et al. 2007. The syndrome of transient epileptic amnesia. *Ann Neurol* **61**(6) 587–598.

Giannantoni, N. M. et al. 2015. Thalamic amnesia mimicking transient global amnesia. *Neurologist* **19**(6) 149–152.

Lee, H. Y. et al. 2007. Diffusion-weighted imaging in transient global amnesia exposes the CA1 region of the hippocampus. *Neuroradiology* **49**(6) 481–487.

Markowitsch, H. J. and Staniloiu, A. 2016. Functional (dissociative) retrograde amnesia. *Handb Clin Neurol* **139** 419–445.

Case: This 75-year-old right-handed woman presented to the clinic for an urgent follow-up due to subacute changes in her speech. She had been diagnosed with Alzheimer disease two years prior, after presenting with a four-year history of progressive memory impairment. Her symptoms were stable until three weeks prior to her follow-up visit, when she became less talkative than usual and started slurring her speech. This was initially attributed to being tired (hectic holidays), but she continued to worsen, prompting an urgent visit to the primary care physician, who ruled out infections and metabolic abnormalities. She eventually plateaued, and the family considered the impaired communication her new baseline. Three days prior to the visit, she had a fall and hit her head. Since then, her speech further declined, and she was having difficulties with dexterity on the right. Although the family was aware she had previous falls, they stated this was the first time she had hit her head.

On exam, she appeared to be tired, and her speech was nonfluent and dysarthric. The remainder of the examination was unchanged overall.

Can You Attribute Her Decline to the Progression of Alzheimer Disease?

Although the rate of decline in Alzheimer disease may accelerate at later stages, the changes here are more rapid than what one would attribute exclusively to advancing neurodegeneration. In cases of subacute worsening of symptoms, a superimposed process should be suspected. Causes of delirium, including infections, such as urinary tract infections or pneumonia, metabolic abnormalities, and medication changes, are the typical categories that require evaluation in the context of an acceleration in functional decline. Given the history of falls, even if they are considered minor and not affecting the head, the possibility of a subdural hematoma or a cerebrovascular event also needs to be considered.

She was evaluated in the emergency department. A CT revealed a large acute-on-chronic subdural hematoma (Figure 13.1). She was immediately taken to the operating room, where the hematoma was drained. After the drainage, her level of alertness and speech improved.

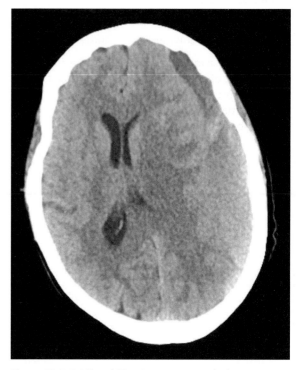

Figure 13.1 Axial head CT in this patient. Note the large acute-on-chronic left subdural hematoma causing mid-line shift.

Discussion

Subdural hematomas (SDH) and other forms of intracranial hemorrhage should be investigated if the more common categories of infection, metabolic changes, and iatrogenic effects cannot explain a subacute decline, particularly if a history of falls can be elicited. The use of antiplatelet or anticoagulation therapies increases the risk for SDH (Baechli et al., 2004). Other findings suggestive of SDH include new-onset headache, seizures, and focal neurologic signs, such as aphasia, hemiparesis, or asymmetric reflexes. Symptoms secondary to SDH may become evident days to weeks after a fall, depending on the rate of hematoma expansion and brain atrophy (Starkstein et al., 2005). Even in cases where there is no report of a fall, a hematoma needs to be assessed, as patients with cognitive impairment may not recall having a fall and there may have been no witnesses.

Importantly, SDH needs to be considered in patients with ventriculoperitoneal shunts who present with worsening headaches and cognitive decline even in the absence of falls. In this case, SDH is considered to result from CSF overdrainage (Marmarou et al., 2005).

Diagnosis: Acute-on-chronic subdural hematoma accelerating Alzheimer disease symptoms

Tip: Marked changes to the rate of decline in neurodegenerative diseases should prompt the investigation of alternative causes, including infection, metabolic abnormalities, changes in medication, and intracranial hemorrhage.

References

Baechli, H., Nordmann, A., Bucher, H. C. and Gratzl, O. 2004. Demographics and prevalent risk factors of chronic subdural haematoma: results of a large single-center cohort study. *Neurosurg Rev* **27**(4) 263–266.

Marmarou, A. et al. 2005. Diagnosis and management of idiopathic normal-pressure hydrocephalus: a prospective study in 151 patients. *J Neurosurg* **102**(6) 987–997.

Starkstein, S. E., Jorge, R. and Capizzano, A. A. 2005. Uncommon causes of cerebrovascular dementia. *Int Psychogeriatr* **17**(Suppl 1) S51–64.

Case: This 67-year-old right-handed woman presented with a 3-year history of memory problems. Her husband reported that she first had difficulty recognizing people, including close family members, such as grandchildren. He also reported she struggled to understand the meaning of words. As an example, she did not cook from recipes anymore, as she could not recognize the ingredients by their names. She had become repetitive and forgetful of recent conversations. However, she was still able to do her own finances, manage medications, and take care of most household chores. A year before her evaluation, her Montreal Cognitive Assessment (MoCA) score was 20/30 due to impairments in clock drawing, naming, phonemic fluency, abstraction, and delayed recall (she did not recall any words freely and recognized four when multiple choices were given). Neuropsychological evaluation revealed predominant language impairment, and brain MRI showed bilateral temporal atrophy (see Figure 14.1). Her presentation was interpreted as early-onset Alzheimer disease, and she was started on donepezil and, later, memantine.

On examination, she was unable to recognize 10 famous people, including the past and current presidents. Severe anomia was evident during the interview, which was more obvious during naming tasks. In addition, there was a loss of word meaning and object knowledge (she could not name nor describe the use of tools). Repetition and grammar were preserved.

Do You Agree with the Diagnosis of Alzheimer Disease?

Her presentation was labeled as memory impairment, as she could not recognize people or understand the use of objects. However, these findings are more suggestive of semantic rather than episodic memory consolidation deficit. The former is associated with anterior and medial temporal lobe atrophy and typical of semantic dementia (SD) most commonly due to TDP-43 proteinopathy; the latter is associated with anterior and posterior hippocampal atrophy and more commonly associated with the classical amnestic syndrome (i.e., impaired memory consolidation) due to Alzheimer disease. In addition, her semantic memory impairment affected specific domains, such as face knowledge (prosopagnosia), which localizes to the nondominant (right) temporal lobe, while language-specific deficits localize to the dominant (left) temporal lobe (Josephs et al., 2008). Considering her right-handedness, this suggested semantic dementia affecting initially the right hemisphere, supported by the asymmetric pattern of atrophy seen on MRI. Deficits in object knowledge and face recognition may occur in Alzheimer disease in advanced stages. This does not fit her presentation, as she is still largely independent in her functioning. Finally, the benefit from cueing indicates the described forgetfulness and repetitiveness is likely due to impaired learning and retrieval strategies, a dysexecutive rather than primary memory consolidation impairment, which also favors semantic dementia, a type of frontotemporal lobar degeneration, rather than Alzheimer disease.

Discussion

Clinical–anatomical correlation remains one of the most important steps in cognitive and behavioral neurology. Given the differential neuronal vulnerability among neurodegenerative disorders, recognizing the neurocognitive and regional brain atrophy patterns can help determine the underlying pathology. Hemispheric lateralization is also relevant. Handedness and language appear to be the two most obvious examples of this hemispheric specialization, likely because they are easier to detect and evaluate. On the other hand, the nondominant (usually right) hemisphere's role in nonverbal aspects of communication and visuospatial abilities is less recognized (Table 14.1). This is relevant as pathologic processes may have regional but not hemispheric selective vulnerability.

In SD, the clinical presentation is dependent on the hemisphere first affected. Lateralizing features are more evident during early stages of the disease; with progression, both temporal lobes become involved and symptoms overlap (Seeley et al., 2005). The dominant (left) hemispheric variant of semantic dementia is associated with semantic deficits described under the semantic variant of primary progressive aphasia (see Case 6), which are usually more evident to the families and easier to detect (Gorno-Tempini et al., 2011). On the other

Table 14.1 Lateralization of cognitive and behavioral functions.

Domain (lobes)	Nondominant (right)	Dominant (left)
Language (frontal and temporal)	Prosody production and comprehension	Phonology, syntax, and semantics; reading and writing
Memory (temporal)	Visual memory	Verbal memory
Gnosis (temporal)	Faces	Words
Praxis (parietal)	Spatial estimation of movements	Skilled motor formulation
Visuospatial (parietal and occipitotemporal)	Awareness of both sensory hemifields Visuospatial perception and constructional abilities	Awareness of contralateral sensory field
Arithmetic (parietal)	Estimation of quantity	Calculation
Executive behavior (frontal)	Inhibition of action	Facilitation of action
Affect (frontal)	Depresses	Elevates

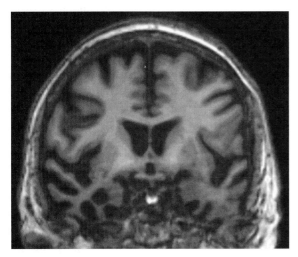

Figure 14.1 Coronal T1-weighted brain MRI in this patient. Note the asymmetric temporal lobe atrophy, affecting the right medial and lateral aspects more than the left.

hand, when the degenerative process predominantly affects the nondominant (right) temporal lobe, deficits in facial processing and changes in behavior emerge (Hodges and Patterson, 2007). Deficits in tasks involving facial processing include impairment in facial recognition, also known as prosopagnosia, as well as impaired ability to recall faces and inability to read face emotions (Josephs et al., 2008). Behavioral changes are characterized by disinhibition, irritability, and rigid thinking (Kamminga et al., 2015). There is lack of consideration for social norms and empathy, which may be related to the inability to process the emotional content of facial expression (Rosen et al., 2002). In addition, patients usually develop compulsions, usually related to words, often using puns (Olney et al., 2017). These changes in behavior make the nondominant (right) variant of semantic dementia difficult to differentiate from the behavioral variant of frontotemporal dementia (bvFTD) (Table 14.2) (Kamminga et al., 2015). This distinction is relevant as it may help identify the underlying pathology. Semantic dementia is more often associated with TDP-43 pathology, whereas sporadic bvFTD is more often associated with tau pathology (Josephs et al., 2009). A thorough history focusing on the early signs of cognitive and behavioral change can help differentiate them. In addition, the different patterns of degeneration can be assessed through structural (e.g., MRI) and functional imaging (e.g., FDG-PET), with involvement of the anterior-medial temporal lobe seen in SD, while frontal and lateral temporal involvement is seen in bvFTD, particularly if the orbitofrontal region is affected.

Diagnosis: Semantic dementia, initially involving the right temporal lobe

Tip: Consider hemispheric lateralization in the diagnosis of cognitive and behavioral impairment. While language and praxis impairments associated with dominant (left) hemisphere may be easier to recognize and evaluate, early nondominant (right) hemisphere deficits, including visuospatial and prosody changes, may be overlooked.

References

Gorno-Tempini, M. L. et al. 2011. Classification of primary progressive aphasia and its variants. *Neurology* **76**(11) 1006–1014.

Table 14.2 Suggested features to discriminate right semantic dementia and behavioral variant FTD

	Right SD	Behavioral variant FTD	Shared impairments
Early signs	Prosopagnosia[a] Topographagnosia[a] Word-finding difficulties	Apathy Executive dysfunction[a]	Disinhibition Reduced empathy
Course of the disease	Prosopagnosia[a] Semantic language deficits[a] Compulsions	Apathy Social withdrawal Preference for sweets[a] Impaired memory Parkinsonism[a]	Dietary changes Decline in self-care
Cognitive evaluation deficits	Language Facial recognition[a] Visual recognition memory	Attention Working memory Executive function	Letter fluency Psychomotor speed

Note: FTD: frontotemporal dementia; SD: semantic dementia.
[a] Highly suggestive.

Hodges, J. R. and Patterson, K. 2007. Semantic dementia: a unique clinicopathological syndrome. *Lancet Neurol* **6**(11) 1004–1014.

Josephs, K. A. et al. 2008. The anatomic correlate of prosopagnosia in semantic dementia. *Neurology* **71**(20) 1628–1633.

Josephs, K. A. et al. 2009. Two distinct subtypes of right temporal variant frontotemporal dementia. *Neurology* **73**(18) 1443–1450.

Kamminga, J. et al. 2015. Differentiating between right-lateralised semantic dementia and behavioural-variant frontotemporal dementia: an examination of clinical characteristics and emotion processing. *J Neurol Neurosurg Psychiatry* **86**(10) 1082–1088.

Olney, N. T., Spina, S. and Miller, B. L. 2017. Frontotemporal dementia. *Neurol Clin* **35**(2) 339–374.

Rosen, H. J. et al. 2002. Emotion comprehension in the temporal variant of frontotemporal dementia. *Brain* **125**(10) 2286–2295.

Seeley, W. W. et al. 2005. The natural history of temporal variant frontotemporal dementia. *Neurology* **64**(8) 1384–1390.

Case: This 58-year-old right-handed man presented with a 3-year history of personality changes and imbalance. His family first noticed he was more withdrawn from social activities and seemed to care less about his appearance. In addition, he was not as affectionate as before and would often make inappropriate comments (e.g., telling people they were overweight). After a recent death in the family, he did not seem to be emotionally affected. More recently, he became more disorganized, which affected his work performance. His gait slowed, and he started to fall frequently. Despite all these changes, he did not seem to be bothered by his symptoms. On neurological examination, he exhibited a resting tremor of the left leg as well as symmetric bradykinesia and upward vertical gaze limitation. His gait was mildly wide-based and unstable, with quick turning (Video 15.1). When asked about family history of neurological disease, he reported his father recently died with Parkinson disease. In addition, out of his five siblings, two older brothers had been diagnosed with dementia and a younger sister with late-onset schizophrenia. His neuropsychological evaluation revealed prominent deficits in executive function, including response inhibition (i.e., ability to suppress inappropriate responses), fluency (i.e., producing words in a limited amount of time), and set-shifting (i.e., switching between different tasks).

How Would You Characterize His Presentation?

The progressive behavioral changes characterized by apathy, lack of empathy, disinhibition and a dysexecutive syndrome suggests the behavioral variant of frontotemporal dementia (bvFTD). His motor presentation with parkinsonism and gaze abnormalities is suggestive of the Richardson syndrome variant of progressive supranuclear palsy (PSP-RS). These two syndromes can overlap in the spectrum of frontotemporal dementia (FTD), which are associated with underlying frontotemporal lobar degeneration (FTLD). In the case of PSP-RS, the underlying pathology is more often a tauopathy. However, other pathologies, including TDP-43 proteinopathy, cannot be ruled out, as they are equally prevalent as tau underlying bvFTD (Josephs et al., 2011).

Does the Family History Offer Any Clues in This Case?

The first impression is that the family history is unrelated to his presentation. However, when contemplating a suspected FTD diagnosis, a genetic etiology needs to be considered. Therefore, obtaining a detailed family history of neurological and psychiatric symptoms is very important. This can be a particular challenge in FTLD, where many different clinical presentations can be seen in families carrying the same mutation (Deleon and Miller, 2018). In addition, the syndromes associated with FTLD are often misdiagnosed. In this case, although the patient reported his father carried a diagnosis of Parkinson disease and his sister of possible schizophrenia, neither underwent formal evaluations nor obtained autopsy confirmation of their diagnoses. It is therefore possible that a bvFTD diagnosis may have been missed in both family members. The family history of parkinsonism, and cognitive and behavioral changes, raises suspicion for a genetic etiology. This plus the presentation with bvFTD and PSP in our patient makes an underlying tauopathy more likely, making MAPT mutation the most likely cause.

A genetic panel including *MAPT*, *GRN* and *C9orf72* genes revealed the presence of a pathogenic *MAPT* mutation.

Discussion

FTD is a group of clinical syndromes associated with the degeneration of the frontal and temporal lobes. They include the behavioral variant of FTD

Video 15.1 Video showing the examination of the patient. Note the symmetric bradykinesia with resting tremor of his left leg and vertical gaze limitation. In addition, he exhibits a mildly wide-based gait with pivotal turning.

Table 15.1 Molecular classification of frontotemporal lobar degeneration and associated genes

	FTLD-tau ~40%	FTLD-TDP ~50%	FTLD-FET ~9%	FTLD-UPS ~1%
Deposited protein	tau	TDP-43	FUS EWS TAF15	Not defined yet[a]
Pathological subtypes	Pick disease CBD PSP GGT AGD	Subtype A Subtype B Subtype C Subtype D Subtype E	aFTLD-U BIBD NIFID	
Associated genes	*MAPT*	*C9orf72* (B and A) *GRN* (A) *VCP* (D) *TARDBP* (all) *SQSTM1* (A and B) *TBK1* (B) *DCTN1#*	*FUS*	*CHMP2B* *UBQLN2*

Note: #TDP-43 pathology for DCTN1 mutation does not match any of the four classic subtypes of TDP-43 classification. AGD: argyrophilicgrain disease; aFTLD-U: atypical frontotemporal lobar degeneration with ubiquitin-positive inclusions; BIBD: basophilic inclusion body disease; C9orf72: chromosome 9 open reading frame 72; CBD: corticobasal degeneration; CHMP2b: charged multivesicular body protein 2B; EWS: Ewing's sarcoma protein; FTLD: frontotemporal lobar degeneration; FUS: fused in sarcoma protein; GGT: globular glial tauopathy; GRN: progranulin gene; MAPT: microtubule associated protein tau; NIFID: neuronal intermediate filament inclusion body disease; PSP: progressive supranuclear palsy; SQSTM1: sequestosome-1; TAF15: TATA-box binding protein-associated factor 15; TARDBP: transactivation response element DNA binding protein; TBK1: TANK-binding kinase 1; TDP-43; transactive response DNA binding protein 43; UPS: UPS: ubiquitin/proteasome system; VCP: valosin-containing protein gene.

*Positive for ubiquitin/proteasome system markers but negative for TDP-43 and FET markers

Source: Adapted from Neumann and Mackenzie (2019).

(bvFTD), semantic dementia (SD) and the nonfluent/agrammatic variant of primary progressive aphasia (nfvPPA). In addition to core cognitive/behavioral features, FTD can be associated with motor syndromes, such as amyotrophic lateral sclerosis, parkinsonism, progressive supranuclear palsy and corticobasal syndrome. Identification of FTD clinically serves the purpose of identifying the cortical region affected and, imperfectly, predicting the underlying pathology. The term frontotemporal lobar degeneration (FTLD) refers to gross and histological (pathological) features. FTLD is currently subdivided into four groups based on abnormally aggregated proteins (Table 15.1).

Up to 10 percent of FTD are inherited in an autosomal dominant pattern, and up to 40 percent of patients have a family history of cognitive impairment (Goldman et al., 2005; Rademakers et al., 2012; Rohrer et al., 2009); bvFTD is most likely to be inherited, followed by nfvPPA, while SD is most often sporadic (Deleon and Miller, 2018). The

genetic mutations most frequently associated with FTD are *C9orf72* gene expansion and *MAPT* and *GRN* mutations, while others, such as FUS, are less frequently found. The list is expected to grow. Identification of these mutations is challenging, as the same primary gene defect can present with a wide range of phenotypes, even within the same family, adding complexity to the diagnostic process. In addition, the presence of FTD in prior generations is often mislabeled as a psychiatric disorder; if dementia was prominent, Alzheimer disease was assumed.

Mutations associated with FTD can also have presentations beyond (and not even including) FTD, such as ALS, PSP, or corticobasal syndrome. Therefore, when considering genetic testing, the first step is to obtain a three-generation pedigree that includes any history of symptoms related to FTD, ALS, other cognitive impairments, psychiatric disorders, parkinsonism, and suicide. However, about 5 percent of symptomatic carriers of mutations associated with FTD have no family history of related

Table 15.2 Select clinical and imaging features of FTLD-associated genetic mutations

	Feature	Genetic mutation associated with
Mode of inheritance	**Autosomal dominant**	*MAPT, C9orf72, GRN, FUS, VCP, CHMP2B, TARDBP, SQSTM1, TBK1, DCTN1*
	X-linked dominant	*UBQLN2*
	Autosomal recessive	*TREM2*
	Anticipation	*C9orf72*
FTD syndrome	**bvFTD**	*All*
	nfvPPA	*MAPT, C9orf72, GRN, TARDBP*, SQSTM1*, TBK1*, CHCHD10**
	svPPA	*MAPT*, C9orf72*, VCP*, TARDBP, TBK1*, TREM2*, CHCHD10**
Neurological features	**Psychosis**	*C9orf72, GRN*, VCP*, FUS*, TREM2*, CHCHD10**
	ALS	*C9orf72, VCP, CHMP2B, TARDBP, SQSTM1, UBQLN2, TBK1, CHCHD10*
	Parkinsonism	*MAPT, GRN, TARDBP, TREM2, CHCHD10*
	Corticobasal syndrome	*GRN, C9orf72*, CHMP2B**
	PSP-like syndrome	*MAPT, GRN*, CHMP2B*, SQSTM1*, UBQLN2**
	Chorea	*C9orf72*
	Cerebellar signs	*C9orf72, TBK1*
	Perry syndrome	*DCTN1*
Nonneurological clinical features	**Paget disease**	*VCP, SQSTM1*
	Myopathy	*VCP, CHCHD10*
	Nasu–Hakola disease (bone cysts)	*TREM2*
	Autoimmune conditions	*GRN*
Imaging features	**Asymmetric atrophy**	*GRN, SQSTM1, TBK1*
	Parieto-occipital atrophy	*GRN, CHMP2B*
	Cerebellar atrophy	*C9orf72*
	Caudate atrophy	*FUS*
	Hippocampal sclerosis	*FUS, TREM2*
	White matter changes	*GRN, TREM2*

Note: Genes with an asterisk represent sporadic reports of the feature. *C9orf72*: chromosome9 open reading frame 72 gene; *CHMP2B*: charged multivesicular body protein 2B gene; *CDCHD10*: coiled-coil-helix-coiled-coil-helix domain-containing protein 10 gene; *DCTN1*: dynactin subunit 1 protein gene; *FUS*: fused in sarcoma protein gene; *GRN*: progranulin gene; *MAPT*: microtubule associated protein tau gene; *PSP*: progressive supranuclear palsy; *SQSTM1*: sequestosome-1 gene; *TARDBP*: transactivation response element DNA binding protein gene; *TBK1*: TANK-binding kinase 1 gene; *TREM2*: triggering receptor expressed on myeloid cells 2 gene; *UBQLN2*: ubiquilin-2 gene; *VCP*: valosin-containing protein gene.

disorders. Other clinical and radiological features may help guide genetic testing, even in patients without a clear family history (Table 15.2).

Diagnosis: Behavioral variant of frontotemporal dementia secondary to MAPT mutation

Tip: Mutations associated with frontotemporal lobar degeneration can exhibit a wide variety of clinical syndromes, even within the same family, including frontotemporal dementia, parkinsonism, and amyotrophic lateral sclerosis.

References

Deleon, J. and Miller, B. L. 2018. Frontotemporal dementia. *Handb Clin Neurol* **148** 409–430.

Goldman, J. S. et al. 2005. Comparison of family histories in FTLD subtypes and related tauopathies. *Neurology* **65**(11) 1817–1819.

Josephs, K. A. et al. 2011. Neuropathological background of phenotypical variability in frontotemporal dementia. *Acta Neuropathol* **122**(2) 137–153.

Neumann, M. and Mackenzie, I. R. A. 2019. Review: neuropathology of non-tau frontotemporal lobar degeneration. *Neuropathol Appl Neurobiol* **45**(1) 19–40.

Rademakers, R., Neumann, M. and Mackenzie, I. R. 2012. Advances in understanding the molecular basis of frontotemporal dementia. *Nat Rev Neurol* **8**(8) 423–434.

Rohrer, J. D. et al. 2009. The heritability and genetics of frontotemporal lobar degeneration. *Neurology* **73**(18) 1451–1456.

CASE 16   Too Many Behavioral Problems for Alzheimer Disease?

Case: A 79-year-old man presented with a 6-year history of worsening gait and balance. He initially complained of heaviness in his legs followed by forgetfulness and a tendency to stumble and fall, initially forward, but he later started falling backward as well. He also manifested word-finding difficulties and trouble with visual navigation. Four years after symptom onset, he developed paranoid ideation and anxiety during a futile trial of levodopa to address the presumptive diagnosis of Parkinson disease. Within months, he became more belligerent, disinhibited, irritable, and uncharacteristically pejorative. He frequently cried and endorsed depression. Word-finding difficulties were compounded by semantic paraphasias ("garage" instead of "cabinet"). He had difficulty locating the food on his plate when eating, particularly if it was located on the left side of the plate. He became wheelchair dependent. His mother had developed dementia in her late seventies. On exam he was alert, but his verbal output was decreased, with hesitations, blocks, semantic and phonemic paraphasias, and palilalia. He exhibited hypomimia, bradykinesia, and rigidity, but no tremor (Video 16.1). A diagnosis of behavioral variant frontotemporal dementia (bvFTD) was made.

What Elements of the History Do Not Fit with the Suspected Disorder?

First, the cognitive deficits preceded the behavioral disturbances by at least four years, suggesting an alternative dementia ultimately manifesting abnormal behaviors. Diagnostic criteria for bvFTD require the behavioral manifestations to be present early in the course of the disease. In addition, his behavioral symptoms were limited to irritability and belligerence, with no evidence of apathy, loss of empathy, perseverations, or dietary changes. Irritability and belligerence may be present in a broad spectrum of

degenerative and nondegenerative dementias, and therefore their presence cannot alone support the diagnosis of bvFTD. Furthermore, the presence of depression highlighted some awareness of his cognitive impairment, unlike bvFTD, where apathy and anosognosia are more common. Finally, even in the late stages, his cognition was affected to a greater extent than his behavior. Dementia with Lewy bodies (DLB) could have been considered as well, given his motor symptoms and the presence of psychosis. However, the absence of hallucinations and cognitive fluctuations made the diagnosis unlikely.

What Features of His Cognitive Dysfunction Could Have Served to Render a More Appropriate Diagnosis?

Evaluating dementia for the first time at an advanced stage presents a challenge. In these cases it is important to obtain a sequential (chronological) history of the timing of onset and course of both cognitive and behavioral impairments. In our patient, his wife had noticed early difficulties with word-finding, memory, and orientation. Unlike typical bvFTD, subsequently language and visuospatial abilities became profoundly affected. Early memory impairment is the most common initial symptom of Alzheimer disease (AD). Impaired word retrieval is a clinical feature of the logopenic variant of primary progressive aphasia (lvPPA), where AD is the most common underlying pathology. Moreover, the presence of hemineglect is suggestive of parietal lobe degeneration, frequently observed in AD. These features should have raised the suspicion for AD.

The patient continued to deteriorate and died within a year of his visit. An autopsy was performed showing high degree of AD neuropathologic changes, with no associated TDP-43 proteinopathy, Lewy bodies, or coexisting tau deposition, suggestive of an underlying tauopathy.

Video 16.1 The examination demonstrates inability to follow commands. He exhibits parkinsonism without tremor and bilateral grasp reflex.

Table 16.1 Main clinical differences between fvAD and bvFTD

	fvAD	bvFTD
Onset of cognitive deficits	Early	Late
Severity of behavioral deficits	Less severe	More severe
Hallucinations and delusions[a]	Common, mild	Rare
Episodic memory	Affected as in classic AD	Preserved until late stages
Executive function	Greatly impaired	Moderately impaired

[a] Very prominent psychotic episodes steer the diagnostic impression into synucleinopathies (most prominently, dementia with Lewy bodies).

Discussion

The presence of behavioral abnormalities may be misconstrued as representing primary rather than secondary phenomenology. The diagnosis of bvFTD is based on a number of behavioral abnormalities (Rascovsky et al., 2011). Using the current diagnostic criteria, the underlying pathology associated with this syndrome is heterogeneous, including tauopathies, TDP-43 proteinopathies and AD (Forman et al., 2006; Josephs et al., 2011). A better understanding of the behavioral and cognitive abnormalities can help predict the pathological process more accurately.

AD affects not only cognition but also mood and behavior, with most AD patients developing neuropsychiatric symptoms during the course of the disease (Steinberg et al., 2008). Besides increasing disability and caregiver burden, neuropsychiatric symptoms herald more rapid progression and shorter survival (Peters et al., 2015). Insidious deterioration of episodic memory is the most common initial symptom of AD and the predominant deficit in the majority of cases. However, it is increasingly recognized that AD may present with different phenotypes. These variants are frequently misdiagnosed (Warren et al., 2012).

In particular, the frontal variant of AD (fvAD) refers to the clinical syndrome of seemingly predominant behavioral and/or dysexecutive deficits with AD as the primary etiology. This variant (or group of variants) of AD may be misdiagnosed as bvFTD, as it may satisfy clinical criteria (Alladi et al., 2007; Forman et al., 2006). However, fvAD is characterized by an earlier and more prominent cognitive deficit compared to bvFTD (Ossenkoppele et al., 2015). Memory is usually impaired to the same degree as classic AD, whereas it tends to be preserved in bvFTD (Ossenkoppele et al., 2015). Conversely, executive function is usually more impaired in fvAD compared to typical early AD and bvFTD, although these may be initially misinterpreted by caregivers as memory impairments (Table 16.1) (Ossenkoppele et al., 2015). In fact, fvAD can present with prominent executive dysfunction (Ossenkoppele et al., 2015).

Behavioral abnormalities and changes in personality represent the most common presentations of bvFTD (Mendez et al., 2013). These deficits tend to be more severe than cognitive impairment (Ossenkoppele et al., 2015). Conversely, behavioral abnormalities in fvAD are less severe and usually appear after cognitive deficits (Ossenkoppele et al., 2015). Finally the presence of hallucinations, delusions, and agitation are suggestive of Lewy body disease and of AD pathology rather than frontotemporal lobar degeneration. (Leger and Banks, 2014; Mendez et al., 2013).

Diagnosis: Frontal variant of Alzheimer disease

Tip: The assessment of a patient with behavioral changes should include a thorough investigation of his cognitive capacities. A preceding and profound degree of cognitive impairment should raise the suspicion for fvAD. The presence of hallucinations, delusions, and agitation suggests underlying AD pathology as well, rather than bvFTD.

References

Alladi, S. et al. 2007. Focal cortical presentations of Alzheimer's disease. *Brain* **130**(Pt 10) 2636–2645.

Forman, M. S. et al. 2006. Frontotemporal dementia: clinicopathological correlations. *Ann Neurol* **59**(6) 952–962.

Josephs, K. A. et al. 2011. Neuropathological background of phenotypical variability in frontotemporal dementia. *Acta Neuropathol* **122**(2) 137–153.

Leger, G. C. and Banks, S. J. 2014. Neuropsychiatric symptom profile differs based on pathology in patients with clinically diagnosed behavioral variant frontotemporal dementia. *Dement Geriatr Cogn Disord* **37**(1–2) 104–112.

Mendez, M. F. et al. 2013. Clinicopathologic differences among patients with behavioral variant frontotemporal dementia. *Neurology* **80**(6) 561–568.

Ossenkoppele, R. et al. 2015. The behavioural/dysexecutive variant of Alzheimer's disease: clinical, neuroimaging and pathological features. *Brain* **138**(9) 2732–2749.

Peters, M. E. et al. 2015. Neuropsychiatric symptoms as predictors of progression to severe Alzheimer's dementia and death: the cache county dementia progression study. *Am J Psychiatry* **172**(5) 460–465.

Rascovsky, K. et al. 2011. Sensitivity of revised diagnostic criteria for the behavioural variant of frontotemporal dementia. *Brain* **134**(Pt 9) 2456–2477.

Steinberg, M. et al. 2008. Point and 5-year period prevalence of neuropsychiatric symptoms in dementia: the Cache County Study. *Int J Geriatr Psychiatry* **23**(2) 170–177.

Warren, J. D., Fletcher, P. D. and Golden, H. L. 2012. The paradox of syndromic diversity in Alzheimer disease. *Nat Rev Neurol* **8**(8) 451–464.

Case: This 57-year old man was brought to the emergency department with a six-month history of episodic jaw pulling and arm flexion and subsequent progressive cognitive decline over this period. Initially rare, the episodes became more frequent. At the time of the hospital admission, he had one nearly every 20–30 minutes. Episodes were brief (three to five seconds) and most often unilateral but could affect either side. He was transiently disoriented with each episode, increasingly even up to a minute after motor signs' termination. Phenytoin, valproate, and clonazepam used during the six-month period prior to admission did not provide any benefit. Initially, he was unimpaired between episodes, but about three months prior to his admission, he was noted to exhibit uncharacteristic slowed thinking and disorganization. He manifested difficulties recalling recent events and repeating stories or questions. He became depressed, withdrawn, and easily irritated. At his initial examination in the hospital, he was observed to have multiple stereotypical episodes (Video 17.1). Bedside Montreal Cognitive Score (MoCA) score was 22/30, with errors in backward digits, serial sevens, phonemic fluency, and delayed recall (he learned three out of five words but was unable to recall any words freely, and only recognized one out of five when multiple choices were given). The rest of the neurological examination was normal. Metabolic panel showed hyponatremia (123 mmol/L). MRI was reported as normal (Figure 17.1). CSF studies showed mild lymphocytic pleocytosis with increased protein, normal glucose, and no oligoclonal bands. EEG showed diffuse slowing, with no ictal changes even during the motor episodes which were subsequently interpreted as myoclonus. Based on the presence of rapidly progressive cognitive impairment with unilateral myoclonus, Creutzfeldt-Jakob disease (CJD) was considered the initial working diagnosis.

Is the Presentation Consistent with CJD?

The evaluation of rapidly progressive dementias can be challenging. Patients are usually evaluated when cognition has already declined significantly, making it difficult to obtain both an accurate sequential history and a comprehensive cognitive evaluation to define the pattern of cognitive impairment. In this case, there were some clinical features pointing away from a diagnosis of CJD. First, CJD is a progressive disorder, and although cognitive fluctuations may be present, intervals of normal cognition are not observed. Moreover, the sustained contractions of his arm and face suggested epilepsy rather than myoclonus, even in the absence of surface EEG abnormalities. The presence of seizures occur in only a minority of CJD cases, usually in later stages (Edler et al., 2009). Additionally, the absence of DWI changes in the cortex or basal ganglia argues against the diagnosis of CJD (Vitali et al., 2011). Finally, the CSF pattern suggested an inflammatory process instead.

In this case, subacute cognitive decline with prominent memory deficits and presence of neuropsychiatric symptoms associated with seizures in the context of an underlying inflammatory process were suggestive of autoimmune limbic encephalitis (LE), even in the absence of EEG and MRI abnormalities. Further support for his diagnosis came from the phenomenology of the episodes observed, which was highly consistent with faciobrachial dystonic seizures (FDBS), a form of LE associated with voltage-gated potassium channel complex (VGKCC) antibodies, more specifically leucine-rich glioma inactivated-1 (LGI1) subtype.

When evaluating a patient with rapid cognitive decline, one of the most important initial steps is to evaluate treatable etiologies, including infectious, toxic, metabolic and autoimmune disorders. In this case, the identification of autoimmune-LE is helpful in prioritizing the workup for rapidly progressive dementia. However, certain conditions may mimic autoimmune-LE and should be considered in the workup (Table 17.1).

Video 17.1 The examination demonstrates two separate episodes of brief arm posturing and ipsilateral face grimacing consistent with faciobrachial dystonia.

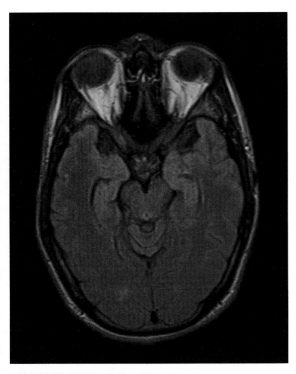

Figure 17.1 FLAIR axial brain MRI in this patient.

Further workup in our patient was negative for human immunodeficiency virus (HIV) and Whipple disease. Herpes and varicella-zoster encephalitis were ruled out in CSF, and 14-3-3 was negative. A serum paraneoplastic panel revealed elevated VGKCC antibodies (4.11 nmol/L), with positive LGI1 protein antibody subtype.

Discussion

Antineuronal antibody-related encephalopathy represents a complex group of autoimmune disorders of the central nervous system. Multiple antibodies and related syndromes have been identified, some with very specific clinical presentations (Table 17.2). The potential response to immunosuppressive treatment and the possible association with underlying cancer warrant a prompt diagnosis. These syndromes can be broadly divided into two groups, depending on the location of the target of the antibody: intracellular or surface. In the first group, the antibodies are not considered to be pathogenic per se but rather an epiphenomenon. Comorbid cancer is common and the response to immunosuppressant therapy poor. On the other hand, in syndromes associated with surface antibodies, underlying cancer is rare, and

Table 17.1 Selected disorders in the differential diagnosis of autoimmune limbic encephalitis

Disorder	Distinctive features
Herpes simplex virus encephalitis	Fever (> 38°C); MRI hemorrhagic lesions in or beyond medial temporal lobes
Human herpesvirus 6 (HHV-6) encephalitis	Most common in immunosuppressed patients
Whipple disease	Systemic symptoms (polyarthralgia and intermittent diarrhea), oculomasticatory myorhythmia
Neurosyphilis	Meningeal signs, uveitis, myelopathy, and MRI findings beyond medial temporal lobe involvement
Metabolic encephalopathy	None neurologically; normal MRI and CSF
Wernicke's encephalopathy	History of alcohol abuse; ophthalmoplegia; ataxia; periventricular hyperintensities; normal CSF
Glioma	Contrast enhancement lesion; usually unilateral
Lymphoma	More common in immunosuppressed patients; contrast enhancement; high ESR, LDH, and beta-2 microglobulin
Amyloid-beta-related angiitis	Positive GRE/SWI microhemorrhages; FLAIR hyperintensities due to edema from inflammation and possibly leptomeningeal enhancement; CSF normal or with mild pleocytosis
Systemic lupus erythematosus	Rash, joint pain
Sjögren's syndrome	Sicca syndrome
Behçet's disease	Recurrent ulcers, uveitis, and polychondritis
Status epilepticus	More common in children and young adults; MRI abnormalities may be present beyond the temporal lobes

Table 17.2 Selected autoimmune encephalopathies

Antibody	Suggestive features	Antibody target	Associated cancer
Antibodies associated with encephalopathies predominantly presenting as LE			
Hu	Encephalomyelitis, sensory neuronopathy	Intracellular	> 95% (SCLC)
Ma2	Hypothalamic failure, narcolepsy-cataplexy, severe rigidity with hypokinesia	Intracellular	> 95% (testicular seminoma)
VGKCC (LGI1)	Seizures (faciobrachial, piloerectile, bradycardic), hyponatremia	Cell surface	5%–10% (thymoma)
GABAb receptor	Seizures, ataxia	Cell surface	50% (SCLC)
AMPA receptor	Psychosis	Cell surface	65% (thymoma, SCLC)
GAD	Stiff person syndrome, ataxia, diabetes	Cell surface and intracellular	25% (thymoma, SCLC)
Antibodies associated with encephalopathies rarely presenting with LE			
CV2 (CRMP5)	Uveitis, retinopathy, chorea, and peripheral neuropathy	Intracellular	> 95% (SCLC, thymoma)
VGKCC (CASPR2)	PNH, Morvan syndrome	Cell surface	20%–50% (thymoma)
DPPX	Diarrhea, rigidity, myoclonus, hyperekplexia, nystagmus	Cell surface	< 10% lymphoma)
GABAa receptor	Intractable seizures, multifocal MRI changes	Cell surface	< 5% (thymoma)
mGluR5	Memory loss, depression, hallucinations, bizarre behavior	Cell surface	70% (Hodgkin lymphoma)
Glycine receptor	Stiff person syndrome, PERM, cerebellar degeneration, optic neuritis	Cell surface	< 20% (thymoma)
Antibodies associated with other encephalopathies			
NMDA receptor	In young women and children; psychiatric, seizures, orofacial dyskinesia, catatonia, autonomic instability, coma	Cell surface	50% (ovarian teratoma)
Dopamine 2 receptor	Dystonia, parkinsonism, oculogyric crises, chorea; MRI basal ganglia abnormalities	Cell surface	0%
GQ1b	Encephalopathy, ataxia, ophthalmoplegia	Cell surface	0%
IgLON5	RBD, OSA, dysarthria, ataxia, chorea	Cell surface	0%

Note: OSA: obstructive sleep apnea; PERM: progressive encephalomyelitis with rigidity and myoclonus; PNH: peripheral nerve hyperexcitability; RBD: REM sleep behavior disorder; SCLC: small-cell lung cancer.

response to immunomodulatory therapy is usually good (Gastaldi et al., 2016).

Voltage-gated potassium channel complex antibodies (VGKCC-ab) were originally thought to target the VGKC itself. However, further research suggested that they actually bind to proteins within the complex, and not the VGKC itself. These binding sites include the leucine-rich, glioma-inhibited 1 (LGI1), contactin-associated protein 2 (CASPR2), and contactin 2 proteins (Irani et al., 2014). Identification of these antibodies is helpful as they are associated with different syndromes and incidence of cancer.

Autoantibodies against VGKC complex have been associated with a spectrum of phenotypes which include limbic encephalitis and seizures, usually associated with LGI1 antibodies, and peripheral nerve hyperexcitability (PNH) and Morvan syndrome, most frequently associated with CASPR2 antibodies

Table 17.3 Syndromes associated with VGKCC-ab

	Limbic encephalitis	Morvan syndrome	Neuromyotonia
Associated antibody	LGI-1	CASPR-2	CASPR-2
Disorientation	++++	++	−
Amnesia	++++	++	−
Seizures	++++	+	−
Insomnia	+	++++	−
Dysautonomia	+	++++	++
Neuromyotonia	−	++++	++++
Abnormal MRI	+++	+	−
Abnormal CSF	++	++	++
Presence of tumor	−	++	++

(Table 17.3) (Irani and Vincent, 2016). Rare presentations include rapidly progressive dementia mimicking CJD, in addition to slowly progressive cognitive decline resembling frontotemporal dementia as well as reports of isolated depression (Geschwind et al., 2008; McKeon et al., 2007; Somers et al., 2011).

LE is the most frequent presentation of VGKCC-LGI1-associated encephalopathy and is more common in men over the age of 50 years, presenting with a combination of rapid cognitive decline and neuropsychiatric changes. There is profound amnesia in the acute phase, affecting anterograde and retrograde components, followed by impairments in executive abilities and language skills (Bettcher et al., 2014; Butler et al., 2014). Neuropsychiatric features, such as apathy, depression and anxiety, typically emerge later in the course but can rarely be the initial presentation (Somers et al., 2011). Mild autonomic dysfunction, including hyperhidrosis and impaired intestinal motility, as well as sleep disorders including insomnia and REM sleep behavior disorder, may be present (Irani and Vincent, 2016; Iranzo et al., 2006). Serum hyponatremia, possibly due to syndrome of inappropriate antidiuretic hormone secretion (SIADH), in the context of LE is a clue to the presence of VGKCC-ab.

Seizures are found in 90 percent of patients with LE associated with VGKCC-LG1, even in the absence of cognitive impairment. Phenomenology may range from focal seizures to status epilepticus. Three seizure semiologies have been strongly associated with VGKC-LG1B: ictal bradycardia, piloerection, and faciobrachial dystonic seizures (FBDS) (Irani and Vincent, 2016). Around 60 percent of patients develop FBDS prior to the onset of cognitive impairment, while another 30 percent develop them in the context of cognitive impairment (Irani and Vincent, 2016). Seizures are brief events involving posturing of the arm and grimacing of the ipsilateral face, with occasional leg involvement. The episodes can occur multiple times a day and affect one side or the other but are not usually simultaneously bilateral. Sensory auras along with postictal confusion and agitation may be present. Surface EEG may not show ictal discharges in a subset of patients, leading to the hypothesis of a subcortical focus (Irani et al., 2011). Seizures are usually refractory to antiepileptic medication but resolve with immunosuppressive therapy.

Imaging abnormalities consist of T2-weighted or FLAIR hyperintensity, but may be normal in up to a quarter of patients (van Sonderen et al., 2016). FDG-PET hypermetabolism in the medial temporal lobe, most often bilateral, occurs, while a similar pattern is observed in the basal ganglia when FBDS are present (Irani and Vincent, 2016). In contrast to most autoimmune encephalitis, the limbic encephalitis associated with VGKCC-LG1B frequently occurs with normal or minimal CSF findings (Leypoldt et al., 2015). However, CSF remains a key step to exclude potential mimics (Irani and Vincent, 2016). Presence of antibodies in serum and CSF are diagnostic in the appropriate clinical setting. Interpretation of positive VGKCC-ab should be done with caution, as low levels are often seen in healthy control populations, ranging between 3.0 percent and 6.9 percent (Dahm et al., 2014). Moreover, VGKCC-ab have been reported in the context of other conditions, including CJD (Newey et al., 2013).

Immunosuppressive therapies often provide significant benefits, including complete resolution of symptoms in some cases (Irani et al., 2014). Normalization of processing speed and executive function with enduring deficits in anterograde memory is the cognitive pattern most commonly observed (Butler et al., 2014). Earlier treatment has been associated with a lower prevalence of residual cognitive impairment, stressing the importance of early diagnosis (Irani and Vincent, 2016). Although the presence of VGKCC-LG1 is in most cases not associated with underlying cancer, screening should be done.

Our patient received methylprednisolone followed by a five-day course of IVIg with complete resolution of his episodes and significant improvement in his cognition. Repeat MoCA (version 2) was 28/30 (missed 2 points in free recall, which resolved with cueing). Whole body PET for cancer screening was normal.

Diagnosis: Limbic encephalitis associated with voltage-gated potassium channel complex antibodies, LGI1 subtype

Tip: When evaluating rapidly progressive dementias, assessment of treatable conditions is a priority. Faciobrachial dystonic seizures, even with normal EEG, are nearly pathognomonic of VGKCC-LGI1 antibody-related encephalopathy.

References

Bettcher, B. M. et al. 2014. More than memory impairment in voltage-gated potassium channel complex encephalopathy. *Eur J Neurol* **21**(10) 1301–1310.

Butler, C. R. et al. 2014. Persistent anterograde amnesia following limbic encephalitis associated with antibodies to the voltage-gated potassium channel complex. *J Neurol Neurosurg Psychiatry* **85**(4) 387–391.

Dahm, L. et al. 2014. Seroprevalence of autoantibodies against brain antigens in health and disease. *Ann Neurol* **76**(1) 82–94.

Edler, J. et al. 2009. Movement disturbances in the differential diagnosis of Creutzfeldt–Jakob disease. *Mov Disord* **24**(3) 350–356.

Gastaldi, M., Thouin, A. and Vincent, A. 2016. Antibody-mediated autoimmune encephalopathies and immunotherapies. *Neurotherapeutics* **13**(1) 147–162.

Geschwind, M. D. et al. 2008. Voltage-gated potassium channel autoimmunity mimicking Creutzfeldt–Jakob disease. *Arch Neurol* **65**(10) 1341–1346.

Irani, S. R. et al. 2011. Faciobrachial dystonic seizures precede Lgi1 antibody limbic encephalitis. *Ann Neurol* **69**(5) 892–900.

Irani, S. R., Gelfand, J. M., Al-Diwani, A. and Vincent, A. 2014. Cell-surface central nervous system autoantibodies: clinical relevance and emerging paradigms. *Ann Neurol* **76**(2) 168–184.

Irani, S. R. and Vincent, A. 2016. Voltage-gated potassium channel-complex autoimmunity and associated clinical syndromes. *Handb Clin Neurol* **133** 185–197.

Iranzo, A. et al. 2006. Rapid eye movement sleep behavior disorder and potassium channel antibody-associated limbic encephalitis. *Ann Neurol* **59**(1) 178–181.

Leypoldt, F., Armangue, T. and Dalmau, J. 2015. Autoimmune encephalopathies. *Ann N Y Acad Sci* **1338** 94–114.

McKeon, A. et al. 2007. Potassium channel antibody associated encephalopathy presenting with a frontotemporal dementia like syndrome. *Arch Neurol* **64**(10) 1528–1530.

Newey, C. R., Appleby, B. S., Shook, S. and Sarwal, A. 2013. Patient with voltage-gated potassium-channel (VGKC) limbic encephalitis found to have Creutzfeldt–Jakob disease (CJD) at autopsy. *J Neuropsychiatry Clin Neurosci* **25**(3) E05–07.

Somers, K. J. et al. 2011. Psychiatric manifestations of voltage-gated potassium-channel complex autoimmunity. *J Neuropsychiatry Clin Neurosci* **23**(4) 425–433.

van Sonderen, A. et al. 2016. Anti-LGI1 encephalitis: clinical syndrome and long-term follow-up. *Neurology* **87**(14) 1449–1456.

Vitali, P. et al. 2011. Diffusion-weighted MRI hyperintensity patterns differentiate CJD from other rapid dementias. *Neurology* **76**(20) 1711–1719.

Contributed by Dr. Marcelo Kauffman and Dr. Sergio Rodriguez Quiroga, Buenos Aires, Argentina

Case: This 29-year-old right-handed woman, diagnosed with schizophrenia at age 21 years, presented with a 3-year history of cognitive decline. Her earliest difficulty was focusing when studying, followed by forgetfulness, both of which affected her performance as a medical student. She ultimately dropped out from school. At the third year of symptoms, her family described her as being disorganized and impulsive. These changes were accompanied by progressive dysarthria and imbalance, with occasional falls.

The earlier diagnosis of schizophrenia, established while she was a medical student, was made because of acute-onset persecutory delusions associated with visual and auditory hallucinations, requiring hospital admission. During that admission she had a generalized seizure, without recurrence since. After failed antipsychotic trials with risperidone, quetiapine, and ziprasidone, she was placed on clozapine, with mild to moderate benefit. She had no family history of neurologic or psychiatric disease. On exam, she was withdrawn and exhibited mild facial dystonia, marked dysarthria, vertical supranuclear gaze palsy, and pancerebellar ataxia (Video 18.1). Montreal Cognitive Assessment (MoCA) score was 21/30 due to impairments in trail making, cube copying, backward digit span, letter A tapping, serial sevens, phonemic fluency, and delayed recall (she learned the five words, recalled two words freely, but recognized the remainder provided multiple choices). Brain MRI was normal.

Could Her Symptoms Be Explained as Part of the Natural History of Schizophrenia? As a Side Effect of Her Medication? Is There an Alternative Explanation?

Both schizophrenia and antipsychotics have been independently associated with a frontal-subcortical pattern of cognitive impairment and movement disorders. However, cognitive decline can precede the first psychotic episode in patients with schizophrenia, with cognitive impairment often stabilizing for years thereafter (Eyler Zorrilla et al., 2000; Harvey, 2012). Atypical antipsychotics have not been associated with cognitive decline in patients with schizophrenia, and some studies have even reported improvement in cognition after treatment with some (such as quetiapine, risperidone, and olanzapine) (Harvey, 2012; Karson et al., 2016). Furthermore, antipsychotics have been associated with dystonia, akathisia, parkinsonism, and tardive dyskinesia, while the latter two may be present in schizophrenia; neither are associated with progressive ataxia, which is the case in this patient (Gervin and Barnes, 2000; Whitty et al., 2009). Importantly, the history of a generalized seizure, the early treatment resistance of her psychosis with presence of visual hallucinations, in addition to the findings of supranuclear gaze palsy and dysarthria on exam, strongly supported an alternative diagnosis to schizophrenia.

What Disorders Should Be Considered in Someone Presenting with Dementia at This Age?

This patient can be classified within the syndrome of young-onset dementia (YOD), defined as progressive cognitive or behavioral decline occurring between the ages of 17 and 45 years (Kelley et al., 2008). The differential diagnosis of YOD can be organized into three groups: early-onset neurodegenerative diseases, adult-onset inborn errors of metabolism (IEM), and age-independent secondary (treatable) causes of dementia (Kuruppu and Matthews, 2013). IEM represent the most common etiology of YOD in patients younger than 30 years (Kelley et al., 2008).

In her case, toxic and basic metabolic panels were unremarkable. The phenomenology (progressive

Video 18.1 The examination demonstrates mild facial dystonia as well as limb dysmetria and gait ataxia.

Table 18.1 Selected inborn errors of metabolism presenting as young-onset dementia

Disease	Presenting features in childhood	Presenting features in adulthood
Urea cycle disorders	Failure to thrive, coma	Vomiting, headache, confusion, stroke-like episodes, ataxia, behavioral changes
Neurotransmitter defects (dopamine synthesis)	Intellectual disability, oculogyric crises, seizures, movement disorders	Focal or generalized dopa-responsive dystonia and/or parkinsonism
Wilson disease	Hepatic failure	Psychiatric signs, tremor, parkinsonism, dystonia
Cerebral glucose transporter (GLUT1) deficiency	Microcephaly, psychomotor delay, epilepsy, dystonia, ataxia	Exercise-induced dystonia, isolated seizures
Mitochondrial disease	Lethargy, hypotonia, failure to thrive, deafness, seizures	External ophthalmoplegia, stroke-like episodes, neuropathy
Adrenoleukodystrophy	Early-onset dementia, visual and hearing impairment, quadriplegia and cerebellar ataxia; leukoencephalopathy is prominent	Psychiatric features, myelopathy, peripheral neuropathy; leukoencephalopathy may be absent or mild
Cerebrotendinous xanthomatosis	Intellectual disability, autism, epilepsy, scoliosis	Dementia, psychiatric changes, cerebellar ataxia, tendon xanthomas

cognitive impairment associated with ataxia and vertical supranuclear gaze palsy) and progression of symptoms, in addition to the evidence of splenomegaly on physical examination, were suggestive of an IEM, more precisely the lysosomal disease Niemann–Pick type C (NPC). Testing with filipin stain on fibroblasts was positive, and genetic testing revealed compound heterozygosity with two mutations affecting the *NPC1* gene (R978C and N1137S), confirming the diagnosis. She was started on miglustat 600 mg/day with improvement in her cognitive, behavioral, and motor symptoms.

Discussion

IEM represents an often overlooked group of mostly autosomal recessive disorders that should always be considered in young adults with cognitive or behavioral impairment. While most IEM present in early childhood with more severe phenotypes, adult-onset forms exhibit more subtle and diverse phenotypes (Table 18.1) (Sedel, 2012). Adult-onset neurological or psychiatric IEM may be underrecognized in the absence of overt systemic involvement (Nia, 2014). Features suggestive of IEM include symptom fluctuation with fasting, exercise, fever, or postprandial status; systemic involvement (e.g., eye or skin problems, organomegaly); and multifocal nervous system involvement (e.g., optic nerves, cerebellum, leukoencephalopathy, and polyneuropathy) (Gray et al., 2000). Some clinical signs are highly suggestive of selected IEM (Table 18.2). In this patient, a previous

Table 18.2 Selected examination findings in patients with young-onset dementia due to inborn errors of metabolism

System	Disorder
Cutaneous	
Angiokeratoma	Fabry disease
Xanthomata	Cerebrotendinous xanthomatosis
Icthyosis	Refsum disease
Ophthalmological	
External ophthalmoplegia	Mitochondrial disease
Supranuclear gaze palsy	Niemann–Pick C (vertical) and Gaucher disease (horizontal)
Macular cherry red spot	Sialidosis, Tay-Sachs disease
Other	
Splenomegaly	Lysosomal diseases
Venous and arterial thrombosis	Homocystinuria

psychiatric diagnosis with the presence of catatonia, visual hallucinations, and psychiatric and cognitive deterioration despite appropriate management all pointed toward an IEM (Demily and Sedel, 2014).

Once the suspicion of IEM is raised, a plethora of differential diagnoses need consideration. A diagnostic approach has been proposed by classifying the different IEM according to the disrupted metabolic process and outlining key characteristics in the presentation of each group (Figure 18.1) (Sedel, 2012). Given the wide distribution and amount of lipids in

Pattern of cognitive impairment	Episodic encephalopathy/psychosis (triggers are common [e.g., fasting, exercise, infections and drugs])		Subacute progression & psychiatric features	Slowly progressive
MRI findings	Stroke-like changes Bilateral basal ganglia lesions	Leukoencephalopathy affecting U-fibers	Metal accumulation in basal ganglia	Leukoencephalopathy sparing U-fibers
Neurologic & systemic findings	Stroke-like episodes Optic neuropathy Seizures Myoclonus Myopathy Cardiomyopathy	Gastrointestinal symptoms during episodes (e.g., nausea, vomiting, and abdominal pain)	Dystonia Parkinsonism Ataxia Choreoathetosis	Seizures Parkinsonism Ataxia Neuropathy Splenomegaly
Inborn error of metabolism	**Energy metabolism defects** Mitochondrial disorders • *MELAS* • *MERRF* • *KSS* Glucose transport disorders • *GLUT-1 transporter deficiency*	**Metabolism intoxication syndromes** Organic acidurias • *Glutaric aciduria* • *Propionic aciduria* Urea cycle disorders • *OTC deficiency* Porphyrias • *AIP*	**Metal storage disorders** Disorders of copper metabolism • *Wilson disease* Disorders of iron metabolism • *PKAN* • *MPAN*	**Lipid storage disorders** Lysosomal storage disorders • *Niemann-Pick type C* • *Gaucher disease* • *MLD* • *Krabbe disease* Peroxisomal diseases • *X-ALD*

Figure 18.1 Classification of inborn errors of metabolism based on pattern of cognitive impairment and MRI findings. The figure is not meant to be exhaustive of all inborn errors of metabolism in adults. Also, as disorders associated with neurotransmitter metabolism are usually not associated with adult-onset cognitive impairment, they are not represented here. AIP: acute intermittent porphyria; KS: Kearns–Sayre syndrome; MELAS: mitochondrial encephalomyopathy, lactic acidosis, and stroke-like episodes; MERRF: myoclonic epilepsy with ragged-red fibers; MLD: metachromatic leukodystrophy; MPAN: mitochondrial membrane protein–associated neurodegeneration; OTC: ornithine transcarbamylase; PKAN: pantothenate kinase-associated neurodegeneration; XALD: X-linked adrenoleukodystrophy.

the nervous system, lipid storage disorders can present with a wide spectrum of clinical phenotypes, including cerebellar ataxia, dementia, psychiatric disorders, epilepsy, spastic paraparesis, polyneuropathy, and leukoencephalopathy (Pastores and Maegawa, 2013; Sedel et al., 2008; Sedel et al., 2008; Staretz-Chacham et al., 2010). They are characterized by a slowly progressive course. Their onset and course are not associated with external triggers. Systemic findings, such as splenomegaly, are highly suggestive of IEM affecting lipid metabolism. Lysosomal storage diseases, which includes Niemann–Pick disease type C (NPC), represent the largest and most common group of disorders within this category.

NPC is an autosomal recessive disease caused by mutations in genes involved in cholesterol esterification and intracellular lipid trafficking, resulting in lipid accumulation in the brain and viscera (Vanier, 2010). Brain pathology is characterized by neuronal and glial lipid storage and tau-positive tangles (Love et al., 1995). Adults usually manifests progressive neurologic or behavioral changes. Psychiatric disorders may be the initial manifestation, remaining isolated for several years. Treatment-refractory psychosis, including paranoid delusions, auditory or visual hallucinations, and behavioral disturbances with aggressiveness, represent the most common psychiatric phenotypes (Josephs et al., 2003; Sedel et al., 2007). Although most NPC patients may have a normal neurologic examination at the time of onset of psychiatric symptoms, abnormalities usually emerge as the disease progresses. Cognitive decline is invariably present, initially affecting executive function, followed by memory impairment (first retrieval, later encoding), progressing to apathy and mutism in later stages (Klarner et al., 2007; Mengel et al., 2013; Yanjanin et al., 2010). Motor impairments include vertical supranuclear gaze palsy, dysarthria and dysphagia (Mengel et al., 2013). Childhood history of gelastic cataplexy is highly suggestive of NPC. Ataxia, usually generalized, represents the most common movement disorder followed by dystonia (usually orofacial), chorea, myoclonus, and parkinsonism (Sevin et al., 2007). Hepatosplenomegaly may be subtle and can provide an important clue to the diagnosis. An NPC Suspicion Index tool is available to aid clinicians in identifying patients with suspicion of NPC (www.npc-si.com/tools) (Wijburg et al., 2012).

The diagnosis of NPC is based on the demonstration of free cholesterol accumulation in cultured fibroblasts from a skin biopsy by filipin staining (Vanier, 2010). Genetic testing for mutations in the *NPC1* (mapped at 18q11) and *NPC2* genes (mapped at 14q24.3) is also available (Vanier, 2010). Miglustat, an inhibitor of glycosphingolipids biosynthesis, has been shown to reduce the progression rate and may stabilize the neurological symptoms (Vanier, 2010).

Diagnosis: Niemann–Pick type C presenting with young-onset dementia and psychosis

Tip: "Primary" psychiatric disorders may be the presenting phenotype of certain dementing neurologic disorders, including adult-onset inborn errors of metabolism. A thorough physical and neurological examination may provide useful clues to guide a diagnostic revision.

References

Demily, C. and Sedel, F. 2014. Psychiatric manifestations of treatable hereditary metabolic disorders in adults. *Ann Gen Psychiatry* **13** 27.

Eyler Zorrilla, L. T. et al. 2000. Cross-sectional study of older outpatients with schizophrenia and healthy comparison subjects: no differences in age-related cognitive decline. *Am J Psychiatry* **157**(8) 1324–1326.

Gervin, M. and Barnes, T. R. E. 2000. Assessment of drug-related movement disorders in schizophrenia. *Adv Psychiatr Treatment* **6**(5) 332–341.

Gray, R. G. et al. 2000. Inborn errors of metabolism as a cause of neurological disease in adults: an approach to investigation. *J Neurol Neurosurg Psychiatry* **69**(1) 5–12.

Harvey, P. D. 2012. Cognitive impairment in schizophrenia: profile, course, and neurobiological determinants. *Handb Clin Neurol* **106** 433–445.

Josephs, K. A., Van Gerpen, M. W. and Van Gerpen, J. A. 2003. Adult onset Niemann–Pick disease type C presenting with psychosis. *J Neurol Neurosurg Psychiatry* **74**(4) 528–529.

Karson, C. et al. 2016. Long-term outcomes of antipsychotic treatment in patients with first-episode schizophrenia: a systematic review. *Neuropsychiatr Dis Treat* **12** 57–67.

Kelley, B. J., Boeve, B. F. and Josephs, K. A. 2008. Young-onset dementia: demographic and etiologic characteristics of 235 patients. *Arch Neurol* **65**(11) 1502–1508.

Klarner, B. et al. 2007. Neuropsychological profile of adult patients with Niemann–Pick C1 (NPC1) mutations. *J Inherit Metab Dis* **30**(1) 60–67.

Kuruppu, D. K. and Matthews, B. R. 2013. Young-onset dementia. *Semin Neurol* **33**(4) 365–385.

Love, S., Bridges, L. R. and Case, C. P. 1995. Neurofibrillary tangles in Niemann–Pick disease type C. *Brain* **118** (Pt 1) 119–129.

Mengel, E. et al. 2013. Niemann–Pick disease type C symptomatology: an expert-based clinical description. *Orphanet J Rare Dis* **8** 166.

Nia, S. 2014. Psychiatric signs and symptoms in treatable inborn errors of metabolism. *J Neurol* **261**(Suppl 2) S559–568.

Pastores, G. M. and Maegawa, G. H. 2013. Clinical neurogenetics: neuropathic lysosomal storage disorders. *Neurol Clin* **31**(4) 1051–1071.

Sedel, F. 2012. Inborn errors of metabolism in adults: a diagnostic approach to neurological and psychiatric presentations. *In* J.-M. Saudubray, G. van den Berghe, and J. H. Walter, eds., *Inborn Metabolic Diseases: Diagnosis and Treatment*. Berlin: Springer, pp. 55–74.

Sedel, F. et al. 2007. Psychiatric manifestations revealing inborn errors of metabolism in adolescents and adults. *J Inherit Metab Dis* **30**(5) 631–641.

Sedel, F. et al. 2008. Movement disorders and inborn errors of metabolism in adults: a diagnostic approach. *J Inherit Metab Dis* **31**(3) 308–318.

Sedel, F. et al. 2008. Leukoencephalopathies associated with inborn errors of metabolism in adults. *J Inherit Metab Dis* **31** (3) 295–307.

Sevin, M. et al. 2007. The adult form of Niemann–Pick disease type C. *Brain* **130**(Pt 1) 120–133.

Staretz-Chacham, O. et al. 2010. Psychiatric and behavioral manifestations of lysosomal storage disorders. *Am J Med Genet B Neuropsychiatr Genet* **153B**(7) 1253–1265.

Vanier, M. T. 2010. Niemann–Pick disease type C. *Orphanet J Rare Dis* **5** 16.

Whitty, P. F., Owoeye, O. and Waddington, J. L. 2009. Neurological signs and involuntary movements in schizophrenia: intrinsic to and informative on systems pathobiology. *Schizophr Bull* **35**(2) 415–424.

Wijburg, F. A. et al. 2012. Development of a suspicion index to aid diagnosis of Niemann–Pick disease type C. *Neurology* **78**(20) 1560–1567.

Yanjanin, N. M. et al. 2010. Linear clinical progression, independent of age of onset, in Niemann–Pick disease, type C. *Am J Med Genet B Neuropsychiatr Genet* **153b**(1) 132–140.

Case: This 66-year-old right-handed woman with a 9-year history of Parkinson disease (PD) presented with worsening anxiety. During the last year, she was noted to worry excessively about different issues (e.g., her grandchildren's safety, her family's wealth), although no recent events could explain these new concerns. She also endorsed depressive symptoms like sadness and lack of energy. Despite the absence of worsening of her motor symptoms, severe apprehension about her condition had emerged. Fluoxetine had been started with mild benefit on her anxiety symptoms. She denied fluctuations in attention and cognitive changes.

On exam, she denied feeling anxious at that moment. She had taken her scheduled dose of levodopa (200 mg QID) 30 minutes before the evaluation and exhibited dyskinesia.

What Strategy Should We Use to Address Her Anxiety?

When neuropsychiatric symptoms emerge in Parkinson disease, the first step is to determine whether they exhibit a continuous or fluctuating pattern. Although both may be secondary to the progression of the disease, the latter is more likely related variations in dopamine levels that may be due to medication effects associated with some long-term PD medication use. It is important to obtain a clear description of the type and severity of neuropsychiatric symptoms and their correlation to the timing of levodopa administration. Somatic features (e.g., palpitations) may differ in nature to psychological symptoms (e.g., excessive preoccupation). Worsening of symptoms earlier between doses suggests a peak-dose phenomenon, while worsening at the end of a dose cycle suggests an OFF phenomenon. The former may be addressed by reducing the dose of levodopa, while in the latter, the dose or its frequency is beneficial. Other strategies to address fluctuations include the use medications (e.g., catechol- O - methyltransferase [COMT] inhibitor), enteral forms of levodopa (i.e., duopa), and deep brain stimulation.

When the patient was asked about the pattern of anxiety and its relationship to levodopa intake, she acknowledged significant worsening of her anxiety 30 minutes before she was due for a dose of levodopa and relief within a half hour after each dose.

Discussion

Dopamine-related nonmotor fluctuations (NMF), which psychiatric and cognitive being two common presentations, are often overlooked, erroneously attributed to motor fluctuations or nondopaminergic degeneration in PD (Martinez-Fernandez et al., 2016; Witjas et al., 2002). NMF are the most usual form of nonmotor fluctuations in PD and can be classified into cognitive, mood, and psychotic (Table 19.1).

Although NMF are often seen in patients with motor fluctuations, the former are not always time-locked nor do they correlate with motor function (Storch et al., 2013). Moreover, some patients present with NMF in the absence of motor fluctuations (Chaudhuri and Schapira, 2009). NMF are more likely to occur during OFF periods, with anxiety and slowness of thinking being the most frequent (Stacy et al., 2005). However, features such as impulsivity, hyperactivity, and a feeling of euphoria that can reach the manic state are observed

Table 19.1 List of selected dopamine-related neuropsychiatric fluctuations and their relationship to the medication state

Domains and symptoms	Distribution in medication state
Cognitive	
• Poor attention	• Predominantly OFF
• Forgetfulness	• Predominantly OFF
• Bradyphrenia	• Predominantly OFF
• Confusion	• Predominantly ON
• Impulsivity	• Predominantly ON
Mood	
• Depression	• Predominantly OFF
• Anxiety	• Predominantly OFF
• Panic attacks	• Predominantly OFF
• Elevation of mood	• Predominantly ON
• Apathy	• Predominantly OFF
• Irritability	• Predominantly OFF
Psychotic	
• Hallucinations	• Predominantly ON
• Delusions	• Predominantly ON
Other	
• Fatigue	• Predominantly OFF

more frequently or exclusively in the ON state (Martinez-Fernandez et al., 2016). Elements of psychosis (e.g., hallucinations) may also represent NMF, usually in the ON state (Bayulkem and Lopez, 2010). Fluctuations in cognition are more complex. While some patients may manifest bradyphrenia and difficulty concentrating in the OFF state which are minimized or eliminated during the ON state, others exhibit these impairments exclusively during the ON state (Martinez-Fernandez et al., 2016).

Finally, other nonmotor fluctuations, including fatigue, autonomic (e.g., orthostatic hypotension), sensory/pain, and sleep impairment (e.g., insomnia), need to be assessed as they may contribute to the presence or severity of NMF (Chaudhuri and Schapira, 2009).

Diagnosis: Parkinson disease with wearing-OFF-related anxiety

Tip: Fluctuating changes in cognition and behavior in Lewy body diseases may arise in the context of or independent of motor fluctuations. Ascertaining its relationship with levodopa dose cycles affords an opportunity to improve these fluctuations by changing the dose or frequency of this medication, among other options.

References

Bayulkem, K. and Lopez, G. 2010. Nonmotor fluctuations in Parkinson's disease: clinical spectrum and classification. *J Neurol Sci* **289**(1–2) 89–92.

Chaudhuri, K. R. and Schapira, A. H. 2009. Non-motor symptoms of Parkinson's disease: dopaminergic pathophysiology and treatment. *Lancet Neurol* **8**(5) 464–474.

Martinez-Fernandez, R., Schmitt, E., Martinez-Martin, P. and Krack, P. 2016. The hidden sister of motor fluctuations in Parkinson's disease: a review on nonmotor fluctuations. *Mov Disord* **31**(8) 1080–1094.

Stacy, M. et al. 2005. Identification of motor and nonmotor wearing-off in Parkinson's disease: comparison of a patient questionnaire versus a clinician assessment. *Mov Disord* **20**(6) 726–733.

Storch, A. et al. 2013. Nonmotor fluctuations in Parkinson disease: severity and correlation with motor complications. *Neurology* **80**(9) 800–809.

Witjas, T. et al. 2002. Nonmotor fluctuations in Parkinson's disease: frequent and disabling. *Neurology* **59**(3) 408–413.

Case: This 68-year-old right-handed woman was evaluated for parkinsonism. Over the prior nine months, she had progressively become more withdrawn from her husband, whom she had been married to for 45 years. Initially, she would intermittently startle when her husband came into the room. Later, she started to sleep in a separate bed and avoided changing her clothes in front of him. When her husband asked her if there was anything wrong, she avoided him without any explanation. She progressively became verbally and physically aggressive toward him, which led to an intervention by her children. When they asked her if there were interpersonal issues between her and their father, she reported that he was not her husband. She acknowledged the resemblance but insisted that he was actually an impostor. Her children's attempts to prove her wrong only made her more agitated. She was taken to the emergency room, where, after ruling out infections, toxic exposures, and stroke, she was given diagnosis of a psychotic disorder and was started on an antipsychotic, risperidone 2 mg daily. While this helped with her agitation, she became slower in her thinking. Her level of attention would fluctuate, and sometimes it appeared as if she were in a daze. In addition, a bilateral hand tremor emerged, and she started to shuffle.

On exam she was oriented to place. Her speech was hypophonic and her discourse tangential at times. She exhibited symmetric bradykinesia, rigidity, and resting tremor. Montreal Cognitive Assessment (MoCA) score was 12/30, due to impairments in trail making, cube and clock drawing, backward digit span, letter-tapping, serial sevens, repetition, phonemic fluency, abstraction, date, and delayed recall. She did not recall any words freely and recognized only two of the words when multiple choices were given.

Can Risperidone Be the Cause of Her Symptoms?

The identification of cognitive slowness and parkinsonism after starting risperidone is suggestive of a drug-induced syndrome. However, the presence of late-onset psychosis should always raise the concern for a neurodegenerative disorder. In this case, the presence of fluctuations and parkinsonism should

raise the concern for dementia with Lewy bodies (DLB). Even if these symptoms appeared to emerge after the medication was started, reviewing the possibility of cognitive changes prior to the alleged onset of symptoms is warranted. In addition, her sensitivity to an antipsychotic medication also supports the suspicion for DLB.

Upon further questioning her family, they reported that she seemed more forgetful and distractible in the past year and that she had stopped cooking, as she could not multitask. Further review of systems revealed a history of dream enactment behavior.

Should We Consider Prosopagnosia in the Differential?

The delusion of a familiar person being replaced by an identical or almost identical double (doppelgänger) whose original has disappeared is known as Capgras syndrome and is most often seen in the context of DLB. Although the double may look familiar, it doesn't typically possess its own name or identity. There is often a sense that the double is threatening, which may provoke violence against the impostor and a search for the "true" person. Capgras may also involve delusions of a duplicate of a familiar place, such as a person's home, which is also perceived as fake, and there is an effort to get to the "real" house. As the most salient feature appears to be the impairment in recognizing a familiar individual, prosopagnosia may be considered in the differential diagnosis. However, in prosopagnosia (apperceptive type) patients are typically able to recognize a face through other modalities (e.g., when the person speaks) and do not harbor the false beliefs of doppelgängers and impostors. In Capgras syndrome, patients can recognize the subject's face, but they do not think it is the person they know.

Discussion

Delusions are defined as fixed beliefs that are not amenable to change in light of conflicting evidence or reason (American Psychological Association, 2013). They are distinguished from hallucinations, which consist of a false perception from any sensory modality (visual, olfactory, etc.). In addition, they

Table 20.1 Selected forms of delusions and their description

Persecutory delusions	Description
Theft	Someone is stealing from the individual
Harm	Someone is monitoring or trying to harm the individual
Infidelity	Individual's spouse is having an affair
Reference	Subtle things occurring in an individual's environment are cues that hold significant meaning
Somatic	Body changes and abnormalities (e.g., sickness, parasitosis, pregnancy)
Grandiose	Grandiose beliefs about oneself (e.g., one's own exaggerated abilities, wealth, or fame)
Control	A person's will, thoughts, and feelings are under the control of external forces
Misidentification syndrome	
Capgras syndrome	Familiar person or place replaced by an identical impostor
Fregoli syndrome	Unfamiliar people or places misidentified as familiar
Cotard syndrome	Patient believe to be dead or part of his/her body has decayed
Phantom boarder syndrome	Someone uninvited living in the patient's home
TV sign misidentification	Events seen on TV are occurring in the patient's current setting
Mirror sign	Not recognizing oneself in the mirror

should be distinguished from delirium, in which the level of alertness or consciousness is impaired, and from confabulations, which are spontaneously spoken fabricated stories but without a fixed belief. Often, confabulatory stories change with multiple interviews, whereas delusions are persistent and reproducible. Moreover, delusions may be classified broadly into two groups. The first one includes persecutory delusions, whereby there is a fixed idea of the subject being targeted, usually with intention of harm. The second group includes misidentification syndromes, where abnormalities in perception lead to delusions (Table 20.1). However, an overlap of features is not uncommon.

The evaluation of new-onset delusions should include a careful assessment of other elements of psychosis, such as hallucinations (visual, auditory, others) and mood changes. Before establishing the diagnosis of a purely psychiatric disorder medical conditions should be ruled out first, particularly when considering late-onset psychosis. This entails ruling out delirium, use or withdrawal of drugs (either elicit or prescribed), decompensation of underlying medical conditions, focal brain lesions (especially right frontal), and cognitive and affective disorders (e.g., DLB, major depressive disorder with psychotic features) potentially associated with a delusional disorder (Reinhardt and Cohen, 2015).

Delusions may occur during the course of all neurodegenerative disorders associated with cognitive impairment. However, the timing of onset along with the associated symptoms may have diagnostic implications. Bizarre delusions, such as those seen in schizophrenia, are rare in neurodegenerative disorders. Delusions tend to occur earlier in dementia with Lewy bodies and later in the course of Parkinson disease (PD) and Alzheimer disease (AD) (Ffytche et al., 2017; Josephs, 2007). Either persecutory delusions or misidentification syndromes may emerge as the first sign of behavioral change in DLB and sometime during the course of the disease in approximately 50 percent of patients (Perini et al., 2016). On the other hand, delusions are rarely present as the initial symptom of PD and AD and are more often observed in the context of moderate to severe cognitive impairment, when the family is already aware of some degree of impairment (Reeves et al., 2012). Persecutory delusions (e.g., theft and infidelity) occur earlier in AD than misidentification delusions, and both increase with dementia severity (Lanctôt et al., 2017). Delusions are not a common feature of frontotemporal lobar degeneration, with the exception of those carrying a C9orf72 abnormal gene expansion (Ducharme et al., 2017). In such cases, delusions (or other forms of psychosis) may be present for up to five years before the patient exhibits typical clinical or imaging features of frontotemporal dementia (Ducharme et al., 2017). Finally, a family history of psychiatric diagnosis may bias toward a purely psychiatric disorder rather than a neurodegenerative process.

Risperidone was discontinued, with improvement in, but not reversal of, her cognitive impairment and parkinsonism. Addition of rivastigmine improved her cognition and substantially attenuated her delusions

Diagnosis: Capgras syndrome in dementia with Lewy bodies

Tip: Delusions, misidentification syndromes, and hallucinations can be presenting features of neurodegenerative dementias, with early appearance in DLB and later appearance in AD.

References

American Psychological Association. 2013. *Diagnostic and Statistical Manual* of *Mental Disorders*. Washington, DC: American Psychological Association.

Ducharme, S., Bajestan, S., Dickerson, B. C. and Voon, V. 2017. Psychiatric presentations of C9orf72 mutation: what are the diagnostic implications for clinicians? *J Neuropsychiatry Clin Neurosci* **29**(3) 195–205.

Ffytche, D. H. et al. 2017. The psychosis spectrum in Parkinson disease. *Nat Rev Neurol* **13**(2) 81–95.

Josephs, K. A. 2007. Capgras syndrome and its relationship to neurodegenerative disease. *Arch Neurol* **64**(12) 1762–1766.

Lanctôt, K. L. et al. 2017. Neuropsychiatric signs and symptoms of Alzheimer's disease: new treatment paradigms. *Alzheimers Dement* **3**(3) 440–449.

Perini, G. et al. 2016. Misidentification delusions: prevalence in different types of dementia and validation of a structured questionnaire. *Alzheimer Dis Assoc Disord* **30**(4) 331–337.

Reeves, S. J., Gould, R. L., Powell, J. F. and Howard, R. J. 2012. Origins of delusions in Alzheimer's disease. *Neurosci Biobehav Rev* **36**(10) 2274–2287.

Reinhardt, M. M. and Cohen, C. I. 2015. Late-life psychosis: diagnosis and treatment. *Curr Psychiatry Rep* **17**(2) 1.

21 Difficulty with Language: When Is It Not Aphasia?

Case: A 70-year-old man had worsening speech over 18 months, with increased effort required to enunciate words. His wife described him as speaking with a monotone voice, and the overall rate of speech was slow. He paused frequently between and in the middle of words, especially during long and complex sentences. He denied problems with finding words, forming sentences, or comprehending spoken or written language. His writing mirrored the slowness in speaking, but there were no abnormalities in its appearance or spelling. On exam, his speech exhibited increased intersegment duration between words, as well as aprosodia. No sound distortions were noticed, except for one false start. Subtle agrammatism was detected early in the interview, though grammar appeared normal during the remainder of the examination (Video 21.1). The rest of his language evaluation and neurological exam was unremarkable. An MRI of the brain demonstrated asymmetric atrophy, predominantly affecting the left premotor cortex.

If the Patient Has Lost Fluency, Would His Be Considered a Nonfluent Aphasia?

Fluency refers to the flow of speech output, and may be affected by multiple factors, including word-finding difficulties, decreased phrase length due to grammatical simplification, or impaired articulation. Although there is no consensus regarding the method to quantitatively evaluate fluency of speech, relying on the number of words per utterance (seven or more words are considered normal) as a parameter is used commonly in clinical practice. However, identifying the nature of the impairment affecting speech output may yield greater diagnostic value than the absolute fluency rate.

Aphasia is defined as a disorder affecting the production or comprehension of language, not caused by sensory or motor impairments (e.g., deafness or articulatory impairment). Although subtle and occasional agrammatism was noticed in our case, his

deficit was predominantly in the motor aspect of speech. However, he does not follow the patterned disorder in articulation and loudness observed in dysarthrias. The phenomenology of his impairment suggests a disorder in speech *motor planning*, known as apraxia of speech (AOS). The slow progression of this type of speech disorder in isolation of any other problem in language is referred to as primary progressive apraxia of speech (PPAOS).

Discussion

The production of speech entails a sequence of cognitive and motor processes (Figure 21.1). The initial step is the selection of the concept chosen to be expressed (e.g., being delighted about a particular situation), followed by the retrieval of the word (or lemma) associated with it (e.g., happy). After the word is chosen, it is modified in order to place the concept in context of the intended message (e.g., unhappy, happiest, happiness), a process known as morphological encoding. This is followed by the selection of phonemes (e.g., h, a, and p), which represent the elemental language units. The sequence of phonemes is translated to a sequence of meaningful sounds known as syllables, which represent the elementary unit of speech (e.g., un-ha-ppy). The proper production of syllables requires very precise motor programming in order to coordinate and sequence appropriately more than 100 muscles. Once the motor program is created, the execution of the motor program relies on the performance of the individual muscle groups.

Apraxia (i.e., inability to perform particular purposive actions) of speech is a motor planning speech disorder characterized by an impaired ability to plan and coordinate the sequential articulatory movements necessary to produce volitional speech sounds (syllables) and the sequencing of muscle movements to produce words. Its symptoms are alterations in articulation, speech segmentation and prosody. Motor planning involves the voiced and unvoiced segments of speech; pauses are as important as spoken elements. Speech apraxia is different from aphasia, given the

Video 21.1 The examination demonstrates slow, monotone speech with pauses between and within words. Subtle agrammatism ("have speaking slowly" and "I would like to know your opinion, what's wrong") is noticed at the beginning. During the description of the cookie theft picture, he said "kitching" when he meant "kitchen."

Video 21.2 Example of a patient with nonfluent variant of primary progressive aphasia. Note the effortful speech.

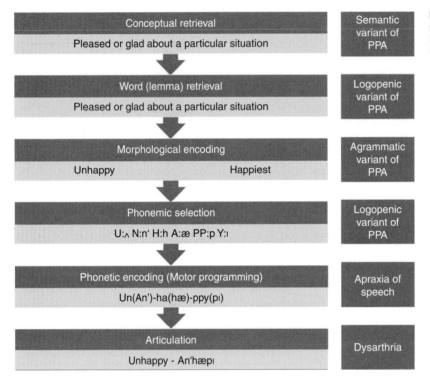

Figure 21.1 An outline of the steps in speech production and its impairments based on the model of Levelt et al. (1999).

preservation of language, and from dysarthria, as the individual movements of phonation are intact (Jung et al., 2013).

AOS manifests with slow, effortful speech and sound production errors (Josephs et al., 2012). Abnormal motor planning leads to nonpatterned sound distortion, which can be perceived as substitutions (for another known syllable or a nonmeaningful sound), additions, or omissions of sounds (Josephs et al., 2012). Impaired syllable production leads to multiple attempts at self-correction, manifesting with false starts, hesitations, and trial and error. A hallmark of AOS is that it becomes more evident with increasing utterance length or word complexity (Gleichgerrcht et al., 2015). Simple words may be articulated without error, while more complex utterances unveil signs of apraxia. The *alternating* motion rates (asking the patient to repeat "puh-puh-puh") may be normal in

apraxia, but *sequential* motion rates (asking the patient to repeat "puh-tuh-kuh") are often poorly sequenced and show a variable pattern of inaccuracies (Josephs et al., 2012). The resulting slower, more cautious speech could be thought of as a compensatory mechanism in order to avoid further errors. Speech is inappropriately segmented, and the intersegment duration within and across words, and also within vowels or consonant segments, is increased (Josephs et al., 2012). Prosody may be affected due to the tendency to stress syllables equally (Josephs et al., 2012). Language is unaffected with preserved productive syntax, semantics, morphology, and comprehension.

However, pure apraxia of speech is relatively rare, and it is not uncommon for AOS to present together with elements of either dysarthria or aphasia, rendering the classification boundaries somewhat blurry. Indeed, differentiating AOS from aphasia

Table 21.1 Speech features present in apraxia of speech and those shared with aphasia and spastic dysarthria

Speech features present only in AOS

- Distorted sound substitutions
- Distorted sound additions
- *Increased sound distortions or distorted sound substitutions with increased utterance length or increased syllable/word articulatory complexity*
- Increased sound distortions or distorted sound substitutions with increased speech rate
- Reduced words per speech breath group relative to maximum vowel duration

Speech features present in AOS and spastic dysarthria

- *Slow overall speech rate*
- *Syllable segmentation within words > 1 syllable*
- Syllable segmentation across words in phrases/sentences
- *Lengthened intersegment durations (between sounds, syllables, words or phrases; possibly filled)*
- Lengthened vowel and/or consonant segments
- *Sound distortions*

Speech features present in AOS and aphasia

- Deliberate, slowly sequenced, segmented, and/or distorted (including distorted substitutions) speech sequential motion rates in comparison with speech alternating motion rates
- Audible or visible articulatory groping; speech initiation difficulty; false starts/restarts
- Inaccurate (off-target in place or manner) speech AMR's (alternating motion rates, as in rapid repetition of "puh-puh-puh")

Speech features present in AOS, spastic dysarthria, and aphasia

- Sound or syllable repetitions
- Sound prolongations (beyond lengthened segments)

Note: Features in italics are the most prevalent among patients with primary progressive apraxia of speech (Josephs et al., 2012).

and dysarthria may be challenging, as they share many features (Table 21.1). A comprehensive and knowledgeable assessment of language and speech is the most important tool to identify the features that characterize this syndrome (Strand et al., 2014). In addition, sound distortions in AOS should not be mistaken with the phonemic paraphasias of aphasic disorders, which are due to incorrect phoneme selection changing the meaning of the word (e.g., "table" instead of "cable," while in AOS you may hear "fuble") but without problems in articulation, speech rate, or prosody seen in AOS. Moreover, the pattern of sound distortion is variable and different from dysarthria, which has a consistent distortion, depending on the muscle groups affected.

AOS may present acutely after a stroke in the left premotor and motor cortices (Graff-Radford et al., 2014). It can also present insidiously as the sole or accompanying feature of a neurodegenerative process, worsening over time, potentially leading to mutism (Duffy and Josephs, 2012). Although AOS is one

of the core diagnostic features of the nonfluent/agrammatic variant of primary progressive aphasia (nfvPPA), the absence of language impairments precludes the diagnosis of PPA (Video 21.2) (Gorno-Tempini et al., 2011). The term *primary progressive AOS* (PPAOS) is preferred when AOS is the initial or predominant manifestation of a neurodegenerative condition, as seen in our case (Josephs et al., 2012). There is increasing evidence that the presence of AOS, as the predominant symptom, even when there is accompanying agrammatism, represents a separate entity from nfvPPA (Josephs et al., 2013).

PPAOS predicts underlying tau pathology, usually distributed in the superior lateral premotor and supplementary motor areas of the left hemisphere (Josephs et al., 2012; Josephs et al., 2006). Progression of the syndrome falls into one of two categories. The first is characterized by predominance of distorted sound substitutions or additions, with insidious language abnormalities evolving over time. The second may remain devoid of aphasic features but becomes associated with parkinsonian features, most often meeting clinical criteria for progressive supra-nuclear palsy (PSP) around five years from symptom onset (Josephs et al., 2014).

In the case of our patient, he returned to the clinic five months after his initial visit and described no significant changes in his speech. This time, his examination showed square-wave jerks, saccadic pursuit, and subtle impairment in corrective downward optokinetic reflexes, which, in association with mild rigidity in the neck, suggested impending PSP.

Diagnosis: Primary progressive apraxia of speech (likely as presenting phenotype of the tauopathy progressive supranuclear palsy)

Tip: Apraxia of speech, which is distinct from both aphasia and dysarthria, is characterized by a slow, effortful speech with increased speech segmentation and sound production errors, particularly in the context of complex and longer words and sentences.

References

Duffy, J. R. and Josephs, K. A. 2012. The diagnosis and understanding of apraxia of speech: why including neurodegenerative etiologies may be important. *J Speech Lang Hear Res* 55(5) S1518–1522.

Gleichgerrcht, E., Fridriksson, J. and Bonilha, L. 2015. Neuroanatomical foundations of naming impairments across different neurologic conditions. *Neurology* **85**(3) 284–292.

Gorno-Tempini, M. L. et al. 2011. Classification of primary progressive aphasia and its variants. *Neurology* **76**(11) 1006–1014.

Graff-Radford, J. et al. 2014. The neuroanatomy of pure apraxia of speech in stroke. *Brain Lang* **129** 43–46.

Josephs, K. A. et al. 2014. The evolution of primary progressive apraxia of speech. *Brain* **137**(Pt 10) 2783–2795.

Josephs, K. A. et al. 2013. Syndromes dominated by apraxia of speech show distinct characteristics from agrammatic PPA. *Neurology* **81**(4) 337–345.

Josephs, K. A. et al. 2012. Characterizing a neurodegenerative syndrome: primary progressive apraxia of speech. *Brain* **135**(Pt 5) 1522–1536.

Josephs, K. A. et al. 2006. Clinicopathological and imaging correlates of progressive aphasia and apraxia of speech. *Brain* **129**(Pt 6) 1385–1398.

Jung, Y., Duffy, J. R. and Josephs, K. A. 2013. Primary progressive aphasia and apraxia of speech. *Semin Neurol* **33** (4) 342–347.

Levelt, W. J., Roelofs, A. and Meyer, A. S. 1999. A theory of lexical access in speech production. *Behav Brain Sci* **22**(1) 1–38; discussion 38–75.

Strand, E. A., Duffy, J. R., Clark, H. M. and Josephs, K. 2014. The apraxia of speech rating scale: a tool for diagnosis and description of apraxia of speech. *J Commun Disord* **51** 43–50.

Case: This 23-year-old woman presented with a four-week history of balance impairment, short-term memory impairment, and irritability. Six weeks prior to her evaluation, she developed Epstein–Barr virus (EBV)-associated infectious mononucleosis, presenting with severe cervical lymphadenopathy and tonsillitis. She was treated with amoxicillin-clavulanate and subsequently prednisone (60 mg a day for 3 days, followed by a 10-day downward titration and discontinuation). Two weeks later, she noted imbalance and a tendency to fall toward the right, along with bilateral loss of hand dexterity. Except for occasional word-finding difficulties, she denied language changes. About the same time, her family noticed she would forget what she had recently been told, particularly lists, and had difficulty driving, damaging three car wheels. Both she and her family reported that her mood was uncharacteristically labile, and she would become easily upset over trivial issues. All of her symptoms peaked at two weeks from onset of imbalance and, since then, had been slowly improving over the subsequent two weeks.

On exam she exhibited symmetric hypotonia, dysdiadochokinesia, dysmetria predominantly in the legs, and gait ataxia (Video 22.1). Her Montreal Cognitive Assessment (MoCA) score was 25/30, with errors in cube copying (Figure 22.1), attention, phonemic (letter) fluency, and sentence repetition. Interestingly, phonemic fluency was markedly impaired (4 in 60 seconds), but semantic fluency was normal (18 in 60 seconds), and she repeated the sentences with subtle grammatical errors (e.g., occasional omissions of auxiliaries such as "be," "have," and "may"). Her affect was consistently elevated (moria; frivolous or childish behavior), and she tended to laugh inappropriately during the exam but did not display any other inappropriate behaviors suggestive of frontal lobe dysfunction or pseudobulbar affect.

How Can We Put This Complex Behavioral Picture Together?

Her brain MRI only showed minimal antero-superior vermal cerebellar atrophy (Figure 22.2). Thus, the absence of parenchymal abnormalities (e.g., masses, white matter changes or strokes), and the subacute presentation of her symptoms after a recent infection with EBV followed by gradual improvement, implicate

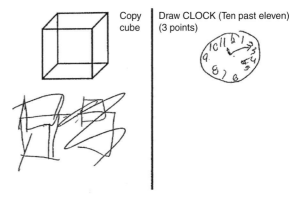

Figure 22.1 Cube copying and clock drawing (from MoCA). Note that in the first attempt, the two cubes are disproportionate. In the second attempt, we can see that the basic elements of the cube are present but not properly organized, suggesting subtle visuospatial deficit. Clock drawing shows slight misplacement of the numbers.

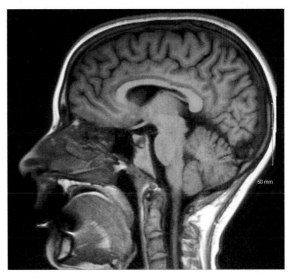

Figure 22.2 T1 sagittal brain MRI in this patient. Minimal atrophy in the anterior and superior aspects of the posterior cerebellar lobe.

a parainfectious (or autoimmune) etiology. Toxic and metabolic etiologies also merit some consideration. Subacute cerebellar ataxia is a rare but well established complication of EBV encephalopathy, even without the systemic features of infectious mononucleosis (Pruitt, 2014).

Video 22.1 The examination shows subtle dysmetria and mild gait ataxia. The patient clarifies that her irritability is not due to her motor impairments.

How Do Her Cognitive and Affective Changes Correlate with Her Cerebellar Features?

The cognitive and affective changes appeared with the cerebellar features she developed shortly after the outbreak of infectious mononucleosis. One may have initially assumed that her affective changes were secondary to the frustration of having to deal with her motor disability. In fact, the cognitive changes emerged independently, and any relationship between motor disability and irritability was denied by the patient (Video 22.1).

The pattern of cognitive and affective changes was reminiscent of what is observed in frontal lobe pathology. Deficient cube drawing could be due to executive problems but may also suggest visuospatial deficits associated with parietal lobe pathology. However, all the cognitive and affective deficits observed can be localized to the cerebellum. Sequelae of parainfectious cerebellitis may suffice to explain all findings.

Discussion

The spectrum of disease caused by EBV is broad and can affect all regions of the central nervous system, with the cerebellum being the most common site (Abul-Kasim et al., 2009). EBV is the most common pathogen associated with acute parainfectious cerebellitis, which may present as a pancerebellar syndrome two to three weeks after the onset of infectious mononucleosis symptoms (Pruitt, 2014). MRI and CSF studies are usually unremarkable, unlike acute EBV meningoencephalitis (Tselis, 2014). Although often self-limiting, motor and cognitive deficits may be permanent (Abul-Kasim et al., 2009; Cho et al., 2013). While steroids are usually not helpful, limited evidence suggests that immunomodulatory treatments, such as plasmapheresis and intravenous immunoglobulin (IVIG), accelerate recovery (Schmahmann, 2004).

Historically, the conception of cerebellar function has been limited to motor and balance control. However, evidence from detailed neuroanatomical investigations, functional neuroimaging studies and neuropsychological assessments of patients with discrete cerebellar lesions suggest the cerebellum plays a role in the modulation of cognitive and affective processes too (Baumann et al., 2015; Manto and Marien, 2015).

Functional disruption of the reciprocal pathways connecting the posterior lobe of the cerebellum, particularly lobules VI and VII, with the prefrontal cortex and temporal, limbic, and parietal association cortices leading to a constellation of cognitive and affective deficits known as the cerebellar cognitive affective syndrome (CCAS) (Koziol et al., 2014). The full expression of the CCAS is characterized by impaired executive function, language deficits, impaired visuospatial processing, and affective dysregulation (Schmahmann and Sherman, 1998). The cognitive deficits associated with cerebellar pathology often do not correlate with motor deficit. Commonly used screening tests like the MoCA or the Mini-Mental State Examination (MMSE) are not sensitive enough to recognize CCSA. When CCAS is suspected, we recommend using the Cerebellar Cognitive Affective/Schmahmann Syndrome Scale, a screening evaluation focusing on the domains affected by the CCAS (Hoche et al., 2018).

Executive function impairments are the most notable and pervasive aspects of the syndrome. Cognitive testing reveals deficits in working memory, phonemic fluency, inhibition, and set-shifting (Tedesco et al., 2011). Patients usually exhibit short-term memory loss mitigated by cueing and demonstrate disruption in mental flexibility (the capacity to shift or switch attention between different tasks or operations typically in response to a change in rules or demands) and perseverative behaviors (Bodranghien et al., 2015). As a result of the impairment in basic executive process, processes that rely on the synergy of executive functions, such as planning and problem solving, are affected (Bodranghien et al., 2015). The reciprocal pathways between the posterior cerebellum and the prefrontal cortex are not involved exclusively in executive functions. A good example of this is memory, where a pattern of impaired free recall with intact recognition is observed, suggesting a retrieval deficit, similar to the one observed with prefrontal disorders and Parkinson disease (Tedesco et al., 2011).

Besides the well-known pattern of cerebellar dysarthria associated with anterior cerebellar lobe dysfunction, apraxia of speech has been described in a number of cases (Marien et al., 2015). Language deficits include decreased verbal fluency, with phonemic (letter) fluency being more affected than semantic (category) naming, in addition to abnormal syntax

Video 22.2 Evaluation four weeks later, showing marked improvement in gait.

resulting in agrammatism and impaired metalinguistic ability (Leggio et al., 2000; Marien and Beaton, 2014). This may lead to a speech pattern characterized by long response latency followed by telegraphic speech, with grammatical errors and inability to understand metaphors, ambiguity, and inferential thinking (Marien et al., 2013).

The role of the cerebellum in visuospatial abilities goes beyond its involvement in oculomotor function. Visuospatial deficits manifest as impaired visual attention and mental representation of spatial relationships between objects, sometimes occasionally presenting as optic ataxia or simultagnosia (Bodranghien et al., 2015). This may be made apparent when attempting to copy or recall visual images (Bodranghien et al., 2015).

Changes in behavior and affect are observed when the posterior vermis and fastigial nucleus are affected and usually resemble milder forms of frontal lobe pathology (Stoodley and Schmahmann, 2010). Patients have difficulty modulating their behavior and may sometimes act in a childlike manner, with disinhibition and impulsive actions (Schmahmann et al., 2007). Affect may be flat or labile, with increased irritability (Bodranghien et al., 2015). A high propensity for laughing and crying, reminiscent of pseudobulbar affect (PBA), has been noted, although the disparity between the emotional experience and expression – a key feature of PBA – is not always present (Bodranghien et al., 2015). Empathy and social cognition may be also impaired (Hoche et al., 2015).

In our patient's case, her symptoms continued to improve without treatment. She was reevaluated four weeks later and was markedly improved. She was able to go back to work and drive, although she admitted a need to be more focused in order to perform optimally. Both she and her family described a return of mood to normal. On examination she exhibited significant improvement of her gait (Video 22.2). An alternative version of the MoCA was done, and she scored 27/30, missing points in rectangle copy, phonemic fluency (eight words in 60 minutes), and sentence repetition (Figure 22.3).

Diagnosis: Cerebellar cognitive affective syndrome due to Epstein–Barr virus–associated parainfectious cerebellitis

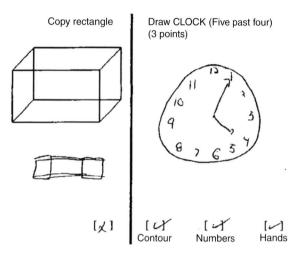

Figure 22.3 Rectangle copying and clock drawing (from MoCA version 2) four weeks later. Note the inability to copy the rectangle, suggesting the persistence of visuospatial deficits. Clock drawing is normal.

Tip: The role of the cerebellum in cognitive and affective modulation should be considered in anyone with cerebellar pathology. Impairments in executive function, language, visuospatial function, and affect or mood from posterior cerebellum resemble milder presentations of cerebral frontal pathology.

References

Abul-Kasim, K., Palm, L., Maly, P. and Sundgren, P. C. 2009. The neuroanatomic localization of Epstein–Barr virus encephalitis may be a predictive factor for its clinical outcome: a case report and review of 100 cases in 28 reports. *J Child Neurol* **24**(6) 720–726.

Baumann, O. et al. 2015. Consensus paper: the role of the cerebellum in perceptual processes. *Cerebellum* **14**(2) 197–220.

Bodranghien, F. et al. 2015. Consensus paper: revisiting the symptoms and signs of cerebellar syndrome. *The Cerebellum* **15**(3) 369–391.

Cho, T. A., Schmahmann, J. D. and Cunnane, M. E. 2013. Case records of the Massachusetts General Hospital: case 30–2013. A 19-year-old man with otalgia, slurred speech, and ataxia. *N Engl J Med* **369**(13) 1253–1261.

Hoche, F. et al. 2015. Cerebellar contribution to social cognition. *Cerebellum* **15**(6) 732-743.

Hoche, F. et al. 2018. The cerebellar cognitive affective/Schmahmann syndrome scale. *Brain* **141**(1) 248–270.

Koziol, L. F. et al. 2014. Consensus paper: the cerebellum's role in movement and cognition. *Cerebellum* **13**(1) 151–177.

Leggio, M. G., Silveri, M. C., Petrosini, L. and Molinari, M. 2000. Phonological grouping is specifically affected in cerebellar patients: a verbal fluency study. *J Neurol Neurosurg Psychiatry* **69**(1) 102–106.

Manto, M. and Marien, P. 2015. Schmahmann's syndrome – identification of the third cornerstone of clinical ataxiology. *Cerebellum Ataxias* **2** 2.

Marien, P. et al. 2013. Consensus paper: language and the cerebellum: an ongoing enigma. *Cerebellum* **13**(3) 386–410.

Marien, P. and Beaton, A. 2014. The enigmatic linguistic cerebellum: clinical relevance and unanswered questions on nonmotor speech and language deficits in cerebellar disorders. *Cerebellum Ataxias* **1** 12.

Marien, P., van Dun, K. and Verhoeven, J. 2015. Cerebellum and apraxia. *Cerebellum* **14**(1) 39–42.

Pruitt, A. A. 2014. Infections of the cerebellum. *Neurol Clin* **32**(4) 1117–1131.

Schmahmann, J. D. 2004. Plasmapheresis improves outcome in postinfectious cerebellitis induced by Epstein–Barr virus. *Neurology* **62**(8) 1443.

Schmahmann, J. D. and Sherman, J. C. 1998. The cerebellar cognitive affective syndrome. *Brain* **121**(Pt 4) 561–579.

Schmahmann, J. D., Weilburg, J. B. and Sherman, J. C. 2007. The neuropsychiatry of the cerebellum – insights from the clinic. *Cerebellum* **6**(3) 254–267.

Stoodley, C. J. and Schmahmann, J. D. 2010. Evidence for topographic organization in the cerebellum of motor control versus cognitive and affective processing. *Cortex* **46**(7) 831–844.

Tedesco, A. M. et al. 2011. The cerebellar cognitive profile. *Brain* **134**(Pt 12) 3672–3686.

Tselis, A. C. 2014. Epstein–Barr virus infections of the nervous system. *Handb Clin Neurol* **123** 285–305.

Case: This 65-year-old right-handed woman presented with a 2-year history of worsening gait and short-term memory impairment. She first noticed slowness in her movements and impaired balance resulting in falls, mostly backward. She tried levodopa titrated to 1200 mg a day with no benefit. Over the previous year, she developed difficulties multitasking and was easily distracted. She endorsed difficulty swallowing and, more recently, urinary incontinence. Her husband noted that she was withdrawn and seemed to have lost interest in hobbies and in social interactions with the family. She denied depression, anxiety, cognitive fluctuations, or hallucinations. She endorsed decreased sense of smell and a history of dream enactment behaviors. On neurological exam, she was easily distractible and tangential. Her speech was hypophonic. Her extraocular eye movements were normal. There was symmetric bradykinesia and distal hand myoclonus when the arms were held outstretched. She was unable to walk unaided (Video 23.1). The Montreal Cognitive Assessment (MoCA) score was 18/30, with impairments in trail making, cube copying, and clock drawing, backward digit span, serial sevens, sentence repetition and delayed recall (she recalled one word freely and recognized the other four when multiple choices were given).

What Elements of Her History and Exam Can Help You with the Diagnosis?

The motor syndrome qualifies as parkinsonism. With the rapid progression of symptoms with early falls and lack of response to levodopa, an atypical parkinsonism appears most likely. Among the neurodegenerative atypical parkinsonisms, two pathologies are more often encountered, alpha-synucleinopathies and tauopathies. Although the motor presentation can be very similar at times, certain elements in the history and presentation favor one rather than the other (Table 23.1). In this case, the presence of dream enactment behaviors, anosmia, and early dysautonomia favors a synucleinopathy. Hand myoclonus was an important motor feature since it can

be a key feature of dementia with Lewy bodies (DLB) and multiple system atrophy, parkinsonian type (MSA-P), but never of Parkinson disease.

Does the Presence of Dementia Rule Out Multiple System Atrophy?

Historically, the presence of early cognitive changes has been held as a feature against the diagnosis of MSA. This was based on early clinico-pathologic studies suggesting a low prevalence of cognitive impairment in MSA (Wenning et al., 1997). However, dedicated neuropsychological assessments often demonstrate cognitive impairment in MSA, with recent reports suggesting its presence in up to 37 percent of pathology-proven cases (Cykowski et al., 2015; Koga et al., 2017). The history accumulated thus far, with prominent dysautonomia but no cognitive fluctuations or hallucinations, favors MSA over DLB.

Discussion

The increasing recognition of cognitive impairment in MSA should temper this as an exclusionary criterion (Stankovic et al., 2014). Dementia has been estimated to emerge after motor and autonomic symptoms, at an average of seven years from the diagnosis of MSA (O'Sullivan et al., 2008). However, case reports indicate that mild cognitive impairment may precede motor and autonomic symptoms. In those MSA patients who survive more than eight years, cognitive impairment eventually develops in almost 50 percent (Brown et al., 2010). The prevalence rates of mild, moderate and severe cognitive impairment in autopsy-confirmed MSA are 22 percent, 2 percent, and 0.5 percent, respectively, but these data are limited by diagnostic criteria that exclude those who present with cognitive impairment (Wenning et al., 1997).

Executive function is the first, predominant, and sometimes only cognitive domain affected in MSA (Stankovic et al., 2014). Manifestations include impaired working memory, response

---

Video 23.1 The examination demonstrates symmetric bradykinesia and distal hand myoclonus when the arms are held outstretched.

Table 23.1 Selected features helpful in the differential diagnosis of atypical parkinsonisms

	Synucleinopathy	Tauopathy
Diseases associated	PD, MSA, DLB	PSP, CBD, FTDP
Motor features	Levodopa-induced dyskinesia Tremor commonly present	Supranuclear gaze palsy Tremor almost always absent
Behavioral features	Hallucinations Cognitive fluctuations	Apathy Disinhibition
Other nonmotor features	Dream enactment behaviors Hyposmia/anosmia Dysautonomia Stridor Head drop	Cortical sensory loss Apraxia of speech

Note: CBD: corticobasal syndrome; DLB: dementia with Lewy bodies; FTDP: frontotemporal dementia with parkinsonism; MSA: multiple system atrophy; PD: Parkinson disease; PSP: progressive supranuclear palsy.

inhibition, phonemic fluency, and set-shifting. Whether attention is separately affected remains a subject of debate. Memory testing demonstrates impairments in learning and retrieval with preserved recognition, suggestive of a frontal-subcortical deficit (Brown et al., 2010; Stankovic et al., 2014). Performance in visuospatial tasks may also be affected (Stankovic et al., 2014). However, whether memory and visuospatial impairments are caused by executive function deficits remains unclear. Language is mostly preserved as reflected by normal performance on repetition and naming to confrontation, even if semantic fluency may be compromised (Stankovic et al., 2014). Ideomotor apraxia is present in about 10 percent of patients (Monza et al., 1998).

There may be differences in cognitive performance between the parkinsonian (MSA-P) and cerebellar (MSA-C) type of MSA (Kawai et al., 2008; Stankovic et al., 2014). While executive impairment is prevalent in both, spontaneous immediate recall deficit is seen in MSA-P, while delayed recall and recognition as well as visuospatial impairment, suggestive of cerebellar cognitive/affective syndrome (see Case 22), are reported to be more frequently impaired in MSA-C (Schmahmann, 2019; Siri et al., 2013; Stankovic et al., 2014). It is important to note that these distinctions in cognitive performance have not been consistently documented and remain controversial (Stankovic et al., 2014).

Behavioral changes are not uncommon in MSA and may affect cognitive performance. Up to 85 percent of MSA patients have at least mild depression, with one-third reported as moderate to severe (Stankovic et al., 2014). Apathy and anxiety are present in 65 percent and 37 percent of patients with MSA (Colosimo et al., 2010; Schrag et al., 2010). Depression is frequently seen in MSA-P, while anxiety is more common in MSA-C (Stankovic et al., 2014).

Diagnosis: Multiple system atrophy, parkinsonian type, with the clinical data available to date; however, future appearance of cognitive fluctuations or hallucinations should steer a diagnostic revision toward dementia with Lewy bodies instead

Tip: The presence of dream enactment behaviors and other nonmotor features can help in the differential diagnosis of atypical parkinsonisms. Early cognitive and behavioral changes should not detract from MSA as a diagnostic consideration.

References

Brown, R. G. et al. 2010. Cognitive impairment in patients with multiple system atrophy and progressive supranuclear palsy. *Brain* **133**(Pt 8) 2382–2393.

Colosimo, C. et al. 2010. Non-motor symptoms in atypical and secondary parkinsonism: the PRIAMO study. *J Neurol* **257**(1) 5–14.

Cykowski, M. D. et al. 2015. Expanding the spectrum of neuronal pathology in multiple system atrophy. *Brain* **138**(Pt 8) 2293–2309.

Kawai, Y. et al. 2008. Cognitive impairments in multiple system atrophy: MSA-C vs MSA-P. *Neurology* **70**(16 Pt 2) 1390–1396.

Koga, S. et al. 2017. Profile of cognitive impairment and underlying pathology in multiple system atrophy. *Mov Disord* **32**(3) 405–413.

Monza, D. et al. 1998. Cognitive dysfunction and impaired organization of complex motility in degenerative parkinsonian syndromes. *Arch Neurol* **55**(3) 372–378.

O'Sullivan, S. S. et al. 2008. Clinical outcomes of progressive supranuclear palsy and multiple system atrophy. *Brain* **131** (Pt 5) 1362–1372.

Schmahmann, J. D. 2019. The cerebellum and cognition. *Neurosci Lett* **688** 62–75.

Schrag, A. et al. 2010. A comparison of depression, anxiety, and health status in patients with progressive supranuclear palsy and multiple system atrophy. *Mov Disord* **25**(8) 1077–1081.

Siri, C. et al. 2013. A cross-sectional multicenter study of cognitive and behavioural features in multiple system atrophy patients of the parkinsonian and cerebellar type. *J Neural Transm* **120**(4) 613–618.

Stankovic, I. et al. 2014. Cognitive impairment in multiple system atrophy: a position statement by the Neuropsychology Task Force of the MDS Multiple System Atrophy (MODIMSA) study group. *Mov Disord* **29**(7) 857–867.

Wenning, G. K. et al. 1997. Multiple system atrophy: a review of 203 pathologically proven cases. *Mov Disord* **12**(2) 133–147.

Case: This 55-year-old left-handed man presented with a 5-year history of progressive behavioral and cognitive decline. Initially, his family noticed he was more withdrawn and irritable. The latter worsened to the point where he exhibited bursts of anger over minor issues. A selective serotonin reuptake inhibitor (SSRI) antidepressant, sertraline, was started and provided moderate benefit. However, over the last two years, he had become distractible, slow in thinking, and increasingly forgetful. These issues affected his performance as an accountant. He had been removed from his responsibilities and assigned to clerical work. He endorsed feeling depressed and anxious. He also complained of a chronic generalized headache, which was moderately relieved by ibuprofen. Before practicing as an accountant, he played rugby professionally for 15 years, retiring at the age of 33. During his career he was knocked unconscious multiple times but reported never having any cognitive or behavioral issues at the time. His father, who also played rugby, was diagnosed with Alzheimer disease at age 65 years.

On exam, he appeared to be anxious, exhibited mild dysarthria, and demonstrated slowness on tapping tasks but without sequential decrement. Neuropsychological evaluation showed deficits in tasks related to executive abilities, with prominent impairments in impulse control (i.e., disinhibition), processing speed, and memory retrieval. Brain MRI showed diffuse atrophy and cavum septum pellucidum. Cerebrospinal fluid evaluation showed amyloid within normal range but elevated p-tau/total tau ratio.

Could This Represent Early Behavioral Variant of Frontotemporal Dementia?

Although he does not meet criteria, it is reasonable to consider bvFTD given the progressive nature of behavioral changes. However, apathy and impulsivity are more often the first behavioral manifestations of bvFTD, compared to the irritability and anger outbursts demonstrated in this case. Moreover, the history of multiple concussions and the complaints of chronic headache suggest trauma, particularly chronic traumatic encephalopathy (CTE), as a possible cause of neurodegeneration. Indeed, although nonspecific, the presence of dysarthria and slowness without bradykinesia in the setting of the cavum septum pellucidum suggest chronic traumatic encephalopathy.

Discussion

Head trauma can have immediate and long-term effects on cognition. Repetitive concussions may lead to a distinct neurodegenerative process, chronic traumatic encephalopathy (CTE). The characteristic pathological findings include aggregation of phosphorylated tau (p-tau) neurons and astrocytes surrounding blood vessels and within the depths of cortical sulci (McKee et al., 2016). Transactive response DNA binding protein 43 (TDP-43) and amyloid pathology may also be present.

Behavioral and cognitive symptoms emerge in the context of a history of repetitive head trauma, with or without loss of consciousness, especially in high-impact sports (e.g., boxing and football) or professions (e.g., military). Symptoms appear after a latency measured in years to decades after the last significant head trauma, with slow progression thereafter. This differs from chronic postconcussion syndrome, where symptoms present immediately after trauma but remain stable (Table 24.1) (Jordan, 2014).

The presentation of CTE includes a combination of behavioral and cognitive symptoms with variable motor symptoms and headache (Figure 24.1) (Montenegro et al., 2014). Behavioral symptoms include emotional lability and explosiveness, occasionally evolving into angry outbursts and violent behaviors. Other behavioral changes include impulsivity and apathy, which may misdirect the diagnosis toward bvFTD if considered in isolation. Depression and anxiety, with suicidal ideation and attempts, are also common. Finally, paranoid behaviors with delusions of persecution or infidelity may be present. Executive cognitive abilities are frequently impaired, along with deficits in simple and divided attention. As the condition progresses memory, language and visuospatial abilities become affected. On examination, variable motor features include dysarthria, psychomotor slowness, parkinsonian features (i.e., bradykinesia, resting tremor, rigidity, and gait impairment), ataxia and upper motor neuron signs. Chronic, dull headache is a common complaint in the early stages (Jordan, 2014).

Table 24.1 Distinctive features of chronic traumatic encephalopathy and chronic postconcussion syndrome

	Chronic traumatic encephalopathy	Chronic postconcussion syndrome
Onset	Insidious	Acute
Progression	Progressive	Nonprogressive
Timing of head trauma	Years before symptoms onset	Immediately before symptom onset
MRI findings	Cavum septum pellucidum Corpus callosum thinning	Normal or nonspecific

Source: Adapted from Jordan (2014).

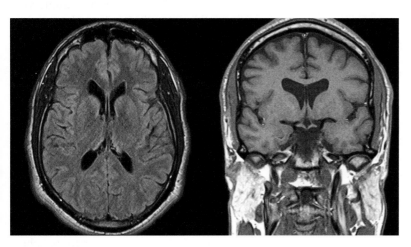

Figure 24.1 T1 axial and coronal brain MRI in this patient. Note the presence of a cavum septum pellucidum as well as mild thinning of the corpus callosum, best appreciated in the coronal section. No other parenchymal abnormalities are present.

Brain imaging may demonstrate callosal, frontal, and hippocampal atrophy. The presence of a cavum septum pellucidum can be considered a diagnostic clue (Bonfante et al., 2018). No established functional neuroimaging or fluid biomarkers exist for CTE and treatment remains symptomatic.

Diagnosis: Cognitive and behavioral changes suggestive of chronic traumatic encephalopathy

Tip: In patients with progressive behavioral and cognitive changes it is critical to ask about past concussive and nonconcussive head trauma and consider the diagnosis of CTE. Special attention needs to be paid to depression and suicidality in CTE patients.

References

Bonfante, E., Riascos, R. and Arevalo, O. 2018. Imaging of chronic concussion. *Neuroimaging Clin N Am* **28**(1) 127–135.

Jordan, B. D. 2014. Chronic traumatic encephalopathy and other long-term sequelae. *Continuum* **20**(6) 1588–1604.

McKee, A. C. et al. 2016. The first NINDS/NIBIB consensus meeting to define neuropathological criteria for the diagnosis of chronic traumatic encephalopathy. *Acta Neuropathol* **131**(1) 75–86.

Montenigro, P. H. et al. 2014. Clinical subtypes of chronic traumatic encephalopathy: literature review and proposed research diagnostic criteria for traumatic encephalopathy syndrome. *Alzheimers Res Ther* **6**(5) 68.

Case: This 65-year-old right-handed man presented with worsening "memory" problems for the past 5 years. He first noticed increasing difficulties with performing previously well-known and simple repairs at home, such as changing a light switch. A neuropsychological evaluation was reportedly normal. More recently, his family noticed declining skills in driving and use of appliances. In addition, performance of other tasks, such as preparing coffee, was affected by pauses and unnecessary steps. More recently, he was forgetful about recent events and unintentionally repetitive. There were no word-finding or navigation difficulties. On exam, he did not appear to be concerned about his impairments and inappropriately joked about them. His speech was fluent with occasional word-finding difficulties. He displayed optic ataxia and oculomotor apraxia, as well as simultanagnosia. In addition, he exhibited ideomotor apraxia with impairments in pantomime (Video 25.1). Montreal Cognitive Assessment (MoCA) score was 10/30 with errors in trail making, cube copy and clock drawing, naming, backward digit span, serial sevens, sentence repetition, phonemic fluency, delayed recall (he did not recall any words freely, and recognized two when multiple choices were given) and orientation to date and day of the week. His brain MRI showed generalized atrophy with greater biparietal atrophy.

How Do You Explain the Normal Neuropsychological Evaluation Earlier in the Course of Symptoms?

The early inability to perform learned tasks as the first sign suggests apraxia was the initial syndrome. In his case, the neuropsychological evaluation did not include an assessment for praxis, which resulted in a report of a "normal" performance and incorrectly reassured the family and delayed clinical evaluation for years. During his exam he exhibited apraxia and other parietal-occipital and temporal-associated deficits (i.e., Balint syndrome, memory impairment, logopenic speech), which suggested Alzheimer disease as the underlying disorder, likely a posterior cortical atrophy variant, especially with early-onset dementia. The initial relative sparing of memory in this variant also likely contributed to the missed diagnosis. However, corticobasal syndrome, dementia with Lewy bodies and prion disease are alternative diagnoses.

Discussion

Apraxia is a deficit of motor programming affecting the performance of a learned skilled movement (Leiguarda and Marsden, 2000). In addition, this impairment cannot be caused by deficits in other cognitive, sensory, or motor domains. In practice, the use of the term *apraxia* is limited to impairments in learned complex movements of the limb or speech. The term *apraxia* is often misused when describing abnormalities of coordinated movements that are either not learned (e.g., "gait apraxia," "oculomotor apraxia," or "eyelid opening apraxia") or whose performance is supported by another cognitive domain (e.g., visuospatial processing deficits lead to dressing and oculomotor apraxia).

While multiple models of limb praxis have been proposed, all of them agree in the prominent role of the left parietal lobe in converting mental images of intended actions into motor execution (Osiurak and Gall, 2012). The left inferior parietal lobe is necessary for the retrieval of the spatial and temporal movement programs needed to carry out the learned skilled movement, known as praxicons. More posterior regions of the left parietal lobe are necessary for the retrieval of the semantic aspects of movements, such as their purpose and use of tools. These praxis centers are activated through different modalities (e.g., visual or verbal) and subsequently activate the motor network. The localization of the disruption of the praxis network is associated with different types of apraxia (Figure 25.1) (Heilman, 2010). However, the network of praxis is still poorly

Video 25.1 The examination demonstrates ideomotor apraxia with impaired pantomime, worse with transitive compared to intransitive gestures. He also exhibits myoclonus.

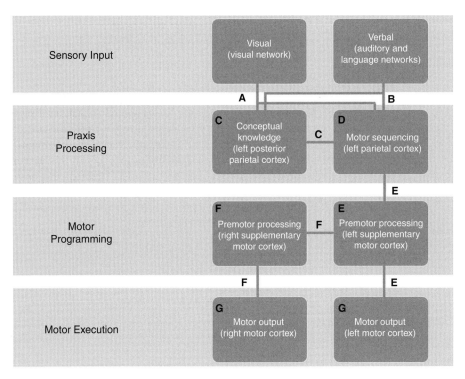

Figure 25.1 Model of praxis and localization damage in apraxia syndromes: (A) dissociation apraxia – visual variant; (B) dissociation apraxia – verbal variant; (C) conceptual apraxia; (D) ideomotor apraxia – parietal variant; (E) ideomotor apraxia – disconnection variant; (F) callosal apraxia; (G) limb-kinetic apraxia.

understood, and other regions of the brain, including subcortical structures, are likely to play a role in praxis.

Apraxia is a deficit often overlooked in neurological disease. Recognition and proper assessment can help in the identification and differential diagnosis of neurodegenerative diseases (Zadikoff and Lang, 2005). For example, given the importance of the parietal lobe in the praxis network, the presence of apraxia can help support a diagnosis of Alzheimer disease, which often affects the parietal lobe, over frontotemporal dementia (Ahmed et al., 2016). In addition, even when the diagnosis is known, the presence of apraxia can be overlooked or attributed to other deficits (e.g., stroke or tremor), missing the opportunity of rehabilitation, which can improve functioning, or caregiver education regarding the need for additional assistance and support.

The assessment of apraxia begins with the evaluation of deficits in other domains that could explain the deficits in learned skill movement performance. These include motor (e.g., paresis, tremor, ataxia), sensory (e.g., primary and higher-level visual deficits), and cognitive (e.g., impaired attention or agnosia) deficits or abnormalities. Once apraxia has been established, a systematic approach to the different aspects of praxis is recommended (Table 25.1). This includes the evaluation of pantomime of transitive (e.g., brushing teeth) and intransitive (e.g., stopping traffic) actions to verbal command, imitation of gestures, gesture knowledge, performance of sequential actions, fine motor movements, and conceptual knowledge of tool use. In addition, transitive gestures are often more affected than intransitive ones in Alzheimer disease compared with other dementias (Mozaz et al., 2006). The pattern of deficits can help define the syndrome and the localization of the deficit (Table 25.1). Most of the current classifications of apraxia include ideational apraxia, which is defined as the inability to perform a task requiring multiple steps in the correct sequence. However, in contrast to other forms of apraxia, the localizing value of ideational apraxia is limited, as it has been reported with frontal damage, suggestive of executive impairment, but also posterior parietal and occipital damage (Heilman, 2010). Treatments primarily involve treatment of the underlying etiologies (e.g., cholinesterase in inhibitors in Alzheimer disease) and rehabilitation strategies, focusing on cueing and strategy training. For the purpose of therapy, understanding the source of the deficit (e.g., praxis instead of memory) can help focus

Table 25.1 Evaluation of apraxia and pattern of impairment in apraxia syndromes

Task	Dis	Con	IM-P	IM-D	Ide	L-K
Pantomime to verbal command Examiner asks the patient to perform transitive (e.g., use scissors) and intransitive actions (e.g., signal someone to come)	+/−	−	−	−	+	+
Imitation of gestures Examiner performs meaningful and meaningless gestures and patient imitates	+/−	+	−	−	+	+
Gesture knowledge Examiner pantomimes meaningful actions and patient names the purpose of the action	+	+	−	+	+	+
Conceptual knowledge Examiner shows tool and patient demonstrates how it is used	+	−	+	+	+	+
Sequential actions Patient pantomimes the performance of a task that requires multiple steps (e.g., prepare a sandwich)	+	+	+	+	-	+
Fine motor movements Patient performs actions that require fine motor movements (e.g., finger tapping)	+	+	+	+	+	−

Note: + normal performance; − impaired performance. Con: conceptual; Dis: dissociation; Ide: ideational; IM-P: ideomotor-parietal variant; IM-D: ideomotor disconnection variant; L-K: limb-kinetic. Callosal apraxia shares the characteristic of ideomotor apraxia – parietal variant but only affects the left limb.

better the strategies and goals. In addition, environmental changes, like removing unsafe objects and simplifying tasks reducing the use of objects, can be considered.

Diagnosis: Possible Alzheimer disease, posterior cortical atrophy variant presenting with ideomotor apraxia

Tip: Impairments in praxis can be the initial sign of a neurodegenerative process. Evaluation for apraxia requires the assessment of different aspects of praxis that can help localize the region affected, with the exception of ideational apraxia. Detection and proper identification of apraxia can help to improve the benefit of rehabilitative therapies.

References

Ahmed, S. et al. 2016. Utility of testing for apraxia and associated features in dementia. *J Neurol Neurosurg Psychiatry* **87**(11) 1158–1162.

Heilman, K. M. 2010. Apraxia. *Continuum* **16**(4) 86–98.

Leiguarda, R. C. and Marsden, C. D. 2000. Limb apraxias: higher-order disorders of sensorimotor integration. *Brain* **123**(Pt 5) 860–879.

Mozaz, M. et al. 2006. Posture recognition in Alzheimer's disease. *Brain Cogn* **62**(3) 241–245.

Osiurak, F. and Gall, D. 2012. *Apraxia: Clinical Types, Theoretical Models, and Evaluation*. Rijeka, Croatia: Neuroscience InTech.

Zadikoff, C. and Lang, A. E. 2005. Apraxia in movement disorders. *Brain* **128**(Pt 7) 1480–1497.

CASE 26   Something Does Not Look Right

Case: This 60-year-old woman presented with a 2-year history of cognitive changes and hallucinations concerning for dementia with Lewy bodies (DLB). She first reported seeing a bright moving circle out of her right visual field. The image was always the same and the episodes lasted 20 seconds. Their frequency increased to five times a day over the course of six months. After each episode, she experienced a headache lasting up to an hour with no associated nausea or photophobia. She had been initially diagnosed with migraine with aura and tried propranolol, verapamil and amitryptline, to no avail. Since starting topiramate six months prior to her evaluation the frequency had reduced to about once a day. However, she felt forgetful, slower in her thinking and had difficulty finding words since initiating topiramate treatment. The development of cognitive impairment in the background of hallucinations had raised the concern for early stages of DLB. However, she denied any motor changes (i.e., parkinsonism) or sleep disturbances (i.e., symptoms of REM sleep behavior disorder).

Her neurological exam was unremarkable, including visual field evaluation. Montreal Cognitive Assessment (MoCA) score was 26/30 due to impairments in backward digit span, phonemic fluency and delayed recall (she recalled three words freely, and recognized one more when multiple choices were given).

Should We Consider Dementia with Lewy Bodies?

Cognitive changes, usually described as word-finding difficulties or as a "brain fog," are common side effects of topiramate (Mula, 2012). In addition, she describes a clear relationship between the onset of her symptoms and the initiation of this medication. Although subjects with DLB can exhibit simple hallucinations, the stereotypical presentation in this case raises the possibility of an epileptic etiology. In addition, over two years, she did not accrue dream enactment behaviors by history or parkinsonian features by exam to support a diagnosis of DLB.

Could We Explain the Hallucinations as Part of the Migranous Syndrome?

Visual phenomena in the context of migraines last minutes to one hour. These usually present as geometric figures (e.g., fortification spectra or teichopsia) or scintillating scotoma. Although these migraine phenomena resemble each other, they are not necessarily identical nor of the same duration between episodes. In addition, her headache did not have additional migranous features, such as nausea or photophobia. Conversely, the phenomenology of epileptic visual hallucinations are often described as brief and with a stereotypical pattern for each individual (Teeple et al., 2009). They can range from brief flashes of light to complex hallucinations depending on the epileptic focus (Elliott et al., 2009a, 2009b). Although patients may describe the episodes as arising from one eye, they represent activity localizing to a visual hemifield. Epilepsy may also lead to illusions where objects may be distorted in size or change shape, referred to as metamorphopsia (Kasper et al., 2010). Finally, occipital seizures are known to be followed by post-ictal headaches (Cianchetti et al., 2013).

A brain MRI revealed a hyperintense lesion affecting her left occipital lobe (Figure 26.1), suggestive of a low-grade glioma. EEG revealed epileptiform activity expressed as occipital transient spikes and sharp waves.

While the antiepileptic effect of topiramate had decreased the frequency of seizures, she was switched to levetiracetam 500 mg twice daily. Her hallucinations disappeared and her cognition improved.

Discussion

Visual perceptual abnormalities are classically divided into two groups: hallucinations and illusions. Hallucinations are visual perceptions in the absence of an external stimulus. In contrast, illusions are misperceptions or misinterpretations of a stimulus in the external environment (Barnes and David, 2001). Translating these clear definitions to clinical practice

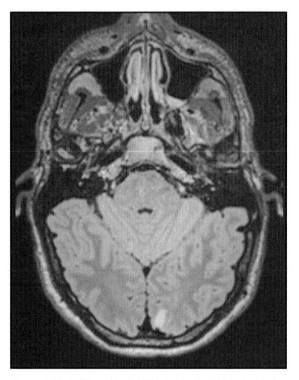

Figure 26.1 FLAIR axial brain MRI in this patient. Note the focal hyperintensity in the left occipital lobe.

may be challenging. In addition, patients may present with both separately or in combination. The mechanisms of visual hallucinations can be broadly divided into three categories: hyperfunction of the visual pathway (epilepsy), sensory deprivation (e.g., Charles Bonnet syndrome) and alteration of arousal or sense of reality (e.g., narcolepsy) (Manford and Andermann, 1998). The phenomenology of visual hallucinations (VH) can be classified as simple or complex. Simple VH can be described as phosphenes (i.e., lights) or photopsias (i.e., geometric structures) and may arise from pathology affecting the eye, usually the retina, or the primary visual cortex. On the other hand, complex VH may arise from sensory deprivation, cortical and subcortical pathology (other than primary visual cortex) and alteration of arousal. VH associated with the ventral (temporal or "what" stream) visual pathway can range from color hallucinations (e.g., hyperchromatopsia) in the more posterior part of the temporal lobe to complex hallucinations of faces, people and landscape with more anterior involvement (Ffytche et al., 2010). Involvement of the dorsal (parietal or "where" stream) pathway is associated with VH

relating motion, like hallucinations of passage or recurrence of past stimulus-induced visual images (palinopsia) (Ffytche et al., 2010). In this patient's case, the description of simple geometic hallucinations suggests occipital involvement.

The conditions associated with VH span different disciplines and need to be interpreted within the context of the patient's presentation (Table 26.1).

VH are reported in neurodegenerative diseases, with a higher prevalence in those with underlying Lewy body pathology, where they can co-occur with hallucinations in other modalities (e.g., auditory) and delusions (Burghaus et al., 2012). These perceptions usually consist of detailed images of unfamiliar people or animals that may be moving or static (Diederich et al., 2009). Hallucinations are generally recurring and brief, although up to one-third of patients report them lasting several hours (Holroyd et al., 2001). Their increased frequency at the end of the day suggest how darkness and reduced vigilance may lower the threshold for their occurrence. They are usually not perceived as frightening, with insight to the hallucinatory nature of these experiences being preserved in nondemented patients and almost two-thirds of patients with dementia early in the course (Fenelon et al., 2000). The emergence of VH is commonly preceded by extracampine hallucinations, usually described as a sense of passage or presence (Bertram and Williams, 2012). Interestingly, there is a higher incidence of epilepsy in DLB and Alzheimer disease (AD), which could be a mechanism to explain the intermittent nature of the hallucinations and psychosis, although more research is needed to support this mechanism (Beagle et al., 2017). VH are a common feature of the Heidenhain (occipital) variant of Creutzfeldt–Jakob disease (CJD) (Gooriah et al., 2014). However, they are uncommon in other neurodegenerative disorders. In Alzheimer disease, VH are present as part of the posterior cortical atrophy syndrome (see Case 10), or in the context of delirium (Linszen et al., 2018). VH are uncommon in frontotemporal lobe degeneration. Their presence in the context of a frontotemporal dementia syndrome should raise the concern for a c9orf72 gene expansion (Boeve et al., 2012).

Diagnosis: Visual hallucinations due to occipital epilepsy secondary to low-grade glioma; topiramate-induced cognitive impairment

Tip: Multiple conditions are associated with visual hallucinations. The phenomenology and duration of

Table 26.1 Select causes of visual hallucinations and their distinct features

Etiology	Distribution	Phenomenology	Duration	Insight	Other features
Lewy bodies pathology	Binocular	*Complex* Unknown people, animals, faces Presence/ Passage hallucinations	Minutes	Depends on degree of cognitive impairment	Visual illusions Parkinsonism Anosmia, dysautonomia REM sleep behavior disorder Cognitive impairment (executive ± visual-spatial)
Peduncular hallucinosis	Binocular	*Complex* Vivid and colorful	Minutes to hours	Usually preserved	Mid-brain pathology (e.g., stroke)
Narcolepsy	Binocular	*Complex* In the context of falling or awakening from sleep	Minutes to hours	Usually preserved	Auditory or tactile hallucinations Sleep paralysis
Epileptic	Contralateral hemifield	*Simple (occipital), complex (temporal) and motion (parietal)* Stereotyped Movement of the image through the visual field	Seconds to two minutes	Preserved	Ictal phenomena (e.g., déjà vu, automatism) Post ictal headache
Migraine	Binocular	*Simple* Scintillating scotoma Teichopsia	Several minutes to an hour	Preserved	Nausea, Photosensitivity Headache
Alcohol withdrawal	Binocular	*Complex* Insects crawling	Hours to days	Impaired	Tactile and auditory hallucination Delirium Dysautonomia
Psychiatric	Binocular	*Complex* People Animals Disruptive	Variable	Impaired	Auditory hallucinations Delusion
Vision loss	Area of vision loss	*Simple or complex* Figures People	Usually minutes; may be continuous	Preserved	Vision loss. No other hallucinations
Retinal pathology	Monocular	*Simple* Flashing light	Seconds	Preserved	Scotoma in area of hallucination Worsened by Valsalva

Note: Simple hallucinations include flashing lights and basic, often bidimensional geometric figures of one or multiple colors. Complex hallucinations include three-dimensional, usually identifiable figures as animals and people. The images may be deformed or disproportionate in size.

hallucinations can be helpful to determine their nature. Stereotyped visual hallucinations lasting less than a minute should raise suspicion for epilepsy.

References

Barnes, J. and David, A. S. 2001. Visual hallucinations in Parkinson's disease: a review and phenomenological survey. *J Neurol Neurosurg Psychiatry* **70**(6) 727–733.

Beagle, A. J. et al. 2017. Relative incidence of seizures and myoclonus in Alzheimer's disease, dementia with Lewy bodies, and frontotemporal dementia. *J Alzheimers Dis* **60**(1) 211–223.

Bertram, K. and Williams, D. R. 2012. Visual hallucinations in the differential diagnosis of parkinsonism. *J Neurol Neurosurg Psychiatry* **83**(4) 448–452.

Boeve, B. F. et al. 2012. Characterization of frontotemporal dementia and/or amyotrophic lateral sclerosis associated with the GGGGCC repeat expansion in C9ORF72. *Brain* **135**(Pt 3) 765–783.

Burghaus, L. et al. 2012. Hallucinations in neurodegenerative diseases. *CNS Neurosci Ther* **18**(2) 149–159.

Cianchetti, C., Pruna, D. and Ledda, M. 2013. Epileptic seizures and headache/migraine: a review of types of association and terminology. *Seizure Eur J Epilepsy* **22**(9) 679–685.

Diederich, N. J., Fenelon, G., Stebbins, G. and Goetz, C. G. 2009. Hallucinations in Parkinson disease. *Nat Rev Neurol* **5**(6) 331–342.

Elliott, B., Joyce, E. and Shorvon, S. 2009a. Delusions, illusions and hallucinations in epilepsy: 1. Elementary phenomena. *Epilepsy Res* **85**(2–3) 162–171.

Elliott, B., Joyce, E. and Shorvon, S. 2009b. Delusions, illusions and hallucinations in epilepsy: 2. Complex phenomena and psychosis. *Epilepsy Res* **85**(2–3) 172–186.

Fenelon, G., Mahieux, F., Huon, R. and Ziegler, M. 2000. Hallucinations in Parkinson's disease: prevalence, phenomenology and risk factors. *Brain* **123** (Pt 4) 733–745.

Ffytche, D. H., Blom, J. D. and Catani, M. 2010. Disorders of visual perception. *J Neurol Neurosurg Psychiatry* **81**(11) 1280–1287.

Gooriah, R. et al. 2014. Visual hallucinations: an unusual manifestation of sporadic Creutzfeldt–Jakob disease termed the "Heidenhain variant." *J Neurol* **261**(11) 2228–2229.

Holroyd, S., Currie, L. and Wooten, G. F. 2001. Prospective study of hallucinations and delusions in Parkinson's disease. *J Neurol Neurosurg Psychiatry* **70**(6) 734–738.

Kasper, B. S., Kasper, E. M., Pauli, E. and Stefan, H. 2010. Phenomenology of hallucinations, illusions, and delusions as part of seizure semiology. *Epilepsy Behav* **18**(1–2) 13–23.

Linszen, M. M. J. et al. 2018. Understanding hallucinations in probable Alzheimer's disease: very low prevalence rates in a tertiary memory clinic. *Alzheimers Dement* **10** 358–362.

Manford, M. and Andermann, F. 1998. Complex visual hallucinations: clinical and neurobiological insights. *Brain* **121** (Pt 10) 1819–1840.

Mula, M. 2012. Topiramate and cognitive impairment: evidence and clinical implications. *Ther Adv Drug Saf* **3**(6) 279–289.

Teeple, R. C., Caplan, J. P. and Stern, T. A. 2009. Visual hallucinations: differential diagnosis and treatment. *Prim Care Companion J Clin Psychiatry* **11**(1) 26–32.

Case: This 44-year-old right-handed woman with 12 years of education presented to the clinic with behavioral changes in the context of abnormal movements. Her husband noticed she became emotionally distant and withdrawn three years prior. Around the same time, she exhibited restlessness and continual movements in her hands, which later spread to her whole body. She was initially thought to be depressed and treated with sertraline (titrated up to 200 mg a day) with no benefit. Within a year of symptom onset, impulsive, inappropriate behaviors emerged (e.g., making comments about other people in public and eating from her husband's plate), accompanied by some delusional thoughts (e.g., thinking her family was trying to hurt her and the government was spying on her).

Her paternal uncle had developed dementia and movements similar to hers. Her father died from amyotrophic lateral sclerosis (ALS) and her mother had unspecified dementia.

On exam, she exhibited a flat affect, along with continual, nonpatterned slow movements of the hands and neck, suggestive of chorea. The remainder of her examination was unremarkable except for hyperreflexia and occasional fasciculations in her legs. Her Montreal Cognitive Assessment (MoCA) score was 24/30, missing points on trail making, cube copying, phonemic fluency and delayed recall (she recalled two words freely, and recognized the other three when multiple choices were given)

General laboratory testing, including lupus panel, was unremarkable. Her brain structural MRI was normal. Genetic testing for Huntington disease (HD) was negative.

What Are the Next Steps in Evaluating Someone with Chorea, Possible Cognitive Decline, and Behavioral Changes Once Huntington Disease Has Been Excluded?

Knowing that the HD testing is normal, focusing on certain aspects of her presentation and history may provide more clues for her diagnosis. First, her cognitive and behavioral presentation with apathy, lack of empathy, and impulsivity are suggestive of the behavioral variant of frontotemporal dementia (bvFTD). In addition, the history of ALS in her family in the context of hyperreflexia and fasciculations raises the concern for a genetic form of motor neuron disease. In familial frontotemporal lobe degeneration presenting with motor neuron disease and chorea, the expansion of the *C9orf72* gene is the most likely etiology.

She was evaluated for *C9orf72* expansion, which was shown to have 3518 GGGGCC repeats, indicative of a pathologic expansion.

Discussion

Huntington disease (HD) represent the most common disorder presenting with the combination of chorea along with cognitive and behavioral changes, especially at the patient's age. The age of onset and speed of progression are correlated with the number of trinucleotide repeats (inversely and directly, respectively). Cognitive impairment usually presents with attention, executive, and visuospatial deficits (Papoutsi et al., 2014). Behavioral changes, including depression, anxiety and personality changes are common as well. Psychosis and aggressiveness are seen at later stages (Eddy et al., 2016).

Up to 7 percent of patients with an HD-like syndrome do not have HD. A growing number of conditions presenting as HD mimics are being recognized. The proper identification of certain clues in the history and examination of the patient can help direct the diagnostic steps (Table 27.1).

The pathologic expansion of the *C9orf72* gene is the most common genetic cause of HD mimics in patients with European ancestry, while *HD-like 2 disorder* is the most common in Africans of sub-Saharan descent (Hensman Moss et al., 2014). In addition, *C9orf72* gene expansion are also the most common genetic cause of frontotemporal lobe degeneration (FTLD) and amyotrophic lateral sclerosis (ALS), which are more common presentations than is chorea. The clinical presentation of *C9orf72* expansion is remarkably heterogeneous, not only between but also within families (Hsiung et al., 2012). Cognitive impairment often presents as bvFTD with disinhibition (which can present as impulsivity),

Table 27.1 Selected conditions presenting as Huntington disease mimics

Disorder	Inheritance (gene)	Distinctive features
C9orf72 repeat expansion	AD (*C9orf72*)	BvFTD features, upper and lower motor neuron signs, psychosis
HDL1	AD (*PRNP*)	Rapid progression
HDL2	AD (*JPH3*)	Affecting Africans of sub-Saharan descent
Spinocerebellar ataxia 17	AD (*TBP1*)	Ataxia, cerebellar atrophy
DRPLA	AD (*ATN1*)	Japanese descent; epilepsy, myoclonus, ataxia
Neuroferritinopathy	AD (*FTL1*)	Asymmetric chorea and dystonia; T2 hyperintensity/T1 hypointensity in basal ganglia; elevated ferritin
Primary familial brain calcification	AD (*SCL20A2, PDGFRB, XPR1*)	Dystonia, parkinsonism; calcification of basal ganglia
Wilson disease	AR (*ATP7B*)	Dystonia, liver disease, Kayser–Fleischer rings
Chorea-acanthocytosis	AR (*VPS13A*)	Tongue-protrusion dystonia, seizures Acanthocytes
McLeod syndrome	X-linked (*XK*)	Similar to chorea-acanthocytosis

Note: AD: autosomal dominant; AR: autosomal recessive; bvFTD: behavioral variant of frontotemporal dementia; HDL: Huntington disease–like.

compulsive behaviors and executive impairment as early features. About a third of carriers manifest language impairment, a nonfluent/agrammatic variant of primary progressive aphasia (Van Mossevelde et al., 2018). Delusional and bizarre behaviors or psychosis, uncommon in bvFTD, should raise concern for a *C9orf72* expansion (Van Mossevelde et al., 2018). In addition, the presence of motor neuron signs, as seen in this case, along with a family history of ALS are clues for *C9orf72* expansion. Besides motor neuron diseases and chorea, parkinsonism and stereotypies have also been described. Brain imaging demonstrates a symmetric atrophy involving primarily the frontotemporal regions, often extending into the parietal and even occipital lobes (Whitwell et al., 2012). In addition, atrophy of the cerebellum and thalamus are more pronounced in *C9orf72* expansion carriers, compared to other genetic causes of FTLD (Bocchetta et al., 2016; Sha et al., 2012).

Diagnosis: Behavioral variant of frontotemporal dementia (bvFTD) and chorea associated with *C9orf72* expansion

Tip: In patients with a HD-like disorder, consider *C9orf72* expansions, especially if associated with motor neuron signs, psychosis, and frontotemporal atrophy.

References

Bocchetta, M. et al. 2016. Patterns of regional cerebellar atrophy in genetic frontotemporal dementia. *NeuroImage Clin* 11 287–290.

Eddy, C. M., Parkinson, E. G. and Rickards, H. E. 2016. Changes in mental state and behaviour in Huntington's disease. *Lancet Psychiatry* 3(11) 1079–1086.

Hensman Moss, D. J. et al. 2014. C9orf72 expansions are the most common genetic cause of Huntington disease phenocopies. *Neurology* 82(4) 292–299.

Hsiung, G. Y. et al. 2012. Clinical and pathological features of familial frontotemporal dementia caused by C9ORF72 mutation on chromosome 9p. *Brain* 135(Pt 3) 709–722.

Papoutsi, M., Labuschagne, I., Tabrizi, S. J. and Stout, J. C. 2014. The cognitive burden in Huntington's disease: pathology, phenotype, and mechanisms of compensation. *Mov Disord* 29(5) 673–683.

Sha, S. J. et al. 2012. Frontotemporal dementia due to C9ORF72 mutations: clinical and imaging features. *Neurology* 79(10) 1002–1011.

Van Mossevelde, S., Engelborghs, S., van der Zee, J. and Van Broeckhoven, C. 2018. Genotype-phenotype links in frontotemporal lobar degeneration. *Nat Rev Neurol* 14(6) 363–378.

Whitwell, J. L. et al. 2012. Neuroimaging signatures of frontotemporal dementia genetics: C9ORF72, tau, progranulin and sporadics. *Brain* 135(Pt 3) 794–806.

Case: This 65-year-old right-handed man presented with a 2-year history of memory complaints. However, he first noticed impaired word recall rather than difficulty recalling events. According to his family, he seemed to know what he wanted to say and compensated with descriptions for lost words but could not produce the intended words. This led to pauses in his speech, which his spouse tried to fill by guessing what he was trying to say. Occasionally, he would "mispronounce" words, making sound errors at a syllabic level. Within the last year, he had become more forgetful, often repeating conversations and missing appointments.

On exam, he exhibited a circumlocutory discourse with pauses between words, especially for nouns. His repetition was impaired, particularly for longer sentences (Video 28.1). Grammar was preserved. He could name 10 out of the 15 items in the short version of the Boston naming test, where he exhibited phonemic paraphasias. The rest of his exam as well as his brain MRI were unremarkable. Prior neuropsychological evaluation was remarkable for impaired free recall (he could recall 3 out 10 items with no benefit from cues).

Do You Consider His Speech to Be Nonfluent?

Fluency is defined by the highest number of words per occasional utterance in a spoken speech sample. In this case, there is a disrupted flow of speech due to pauses between words associated with impaired word retrieval but not an impairment to link words into sentences. During his interview, he was able to link five to seven words per utterance, which is considered normal fluency. In addition, his speech did not appear to be effortful nor involve alterations in prosody, articulation, or grammar (Video 28.2). Rather than nonfluent, this pattern of speech is considered logopenic. In nonfluent speech, articulation and naming are effortful, with difficulties emerging in the middle of the word, particularly in those with multiple syllables. Due to impaired grammar, words cannot be linked together in a sentence, sentences lack function words, and errors are made in inflections, all leading to a telegraphic speech pattern and impaired word

repetition. In both cases paraphasias can be present. However, in logopenic speech, these are largely due to the selection of an incorrect syllable, correctly enunciated (e.g., "pable" instead of "table," also known as phonemic paraphasias). In nonfluent speech, conversely, articulatory errors can lead to mispronunciation of the correct syllable, also known as phonetic paraphasias, which are often associated with false starts. Articulatory errors are a feature of apraxia of speech.

Can He Be Classified as a Logopenic Variant of Primary Progressive Aphasia Even in the Setting of Memory Impairment?

One of the main goals of establishing the specific language syndrome is to aid in determining the underlying pathology. In this case, classifying the speech disorder as the logopenic variant of primary progressive aphasia (lvPPA) allows an assumption that the underlying pathology is likely Alzheimer disease (AD). The diagnosis of PPA requires language to be the first and most affected domain. However, other domains can be affected as the disease progresses, such as, in this case, impairments in memory consistent with those seen in AD.

Discussion

The logopenic variant of primary progressive aphasia (lvPPA) is a syndrome associated with the degeneration of the temporoparietal junction in the dominant hemisphere. This region contains areas involved in activating phonological representations linking verbal semantic stores to language output (Rohrer et al., 2008). In addition, it contains the phonological loop, a key area of the working memory network (Gorno-Tempini et al., 2008). The phonological loop serves as a buffer, in which phonological memory traces are held over a period of few seconds and sustained through articulatory rehearsal (Baddeley and Hitch, 2019). In language, this translates to longer words and sentences. Alzheimer disease is the most common pathology associated with lvPPA (Table 28.1). The language disturbances reported in lvPPA closely

Table 28.1 Clinical and imaging criteria of the three variants of primary progressive aphasia

	svPPA	nfvPPA	lvPPA
Clinical criteria	*Both of:*	*At least one of:*	*Both of:*
	Impaired confrontation naming	Agrammatism in language production	Impaired single-word retrieval in spontaneous speech and naming
	Impaired single-word comprehension	Effortful, halting speech with inconsistent speech sound errors, and distortions (speech apraxia)	Impaired repetition of sentences and phrases
	At least three of:	*At least two of:*	*At least three of:*
	Impaired object knowledge, particularly for low-frequency or low-familiarity items	Impaired comprehension of syntactically complex sentences	Speech (phonologic) errors in spontaneous speech and naming
	Surface dyslexia or dysgraphia	Spared single-word comprehension	Spared single-word comprehension and object knowledge
	Spared repetition	Spared object knowledge	Spared motor speech
	Spared speech production (grammar and motor speech)		Absence of frank agrammatism
Area affected[a]	Anterio-medial temporal lobe	Left posterior fronto-insular region	Left posterior peri-sylvian and parietal region
Most frequent pathology	TDP-43 Type C proteinopathy	Tauopathy	Alzheimer disease

Note: lvPPA: logopenic variant of primary progressive aphasia; nfvPPA: nonfluent/agrammatic variant of primary progressive aphasia; svPPA: semantic variant of primary progressive aphasia.

[a] Can be evaluated by atrophy in MRI or hypometabolism in PET/SPECT.

resemble those that generally develop during the progression of the more common presentation of AD, the amnestic variant (Snowden et al., 2007).

Patients typically exhibit an irregular rate of speech, mainly due to pauses while attempting to retrieve words (Marshall et al., 2018). Sentence repetition is characteristically impaired, affecting disproportionately long sentences with words that occur infrequently in spoken language. For example, repetition of "The phantom soared across the foggy heath" is more likely to be impaired than "I went to the store to buy a loaf of bread." Generally, phonemic paraphasias can be observed during spontaneous speech or reading. The inability to retrieve the correct phoneme can lead to neologisms or jargon (e.g., "stunabler" instead of "computer") (Marshall et al., 2018). Confrontation naming may be impaired. Self-generated word searches during spontaneous speech are more likely to result in paraphasic errors, but visual cues from confrontation naming typically reduce the work for retrieving phonemic sound patterns. Grammar is largely preserved along with articulation and prosody, features that help distinguishing lvPPA from the nonfluent variant of PPA (Video 28.3) (Wilson et al., 2010). However, due to the deficit of the phonological loop, impairments of understanding long sentences can be

Video 28.1 The examination demonstrates circumlocutory discourse with long sentences. Phonemic paraphasia when trying to name "cacti" is shown. Repetition is impaired.

Video 28.2 Examination of a patient with nfvPPA. Note the effortful, telegraphic speech with impaired grammar.

Video 28.3 Video showing description of the Boston Cookie Jar Theft Picture by patients with different impairments in language. First is lvPPA (the present case) exhibiting pauses between words and difficulty with names. Second is nfvPPA with effortful, telegraphic speech and simplified grammar. Third is the semantic variant of primary progressive aphasia, exhibiting fluent speech with agnosia. Last is behavioral variant of frontotemporal dementia, manifesting a fluent but concise speech with inappropriate comments.

Table 28.2 Clinical features of the three different variants of primary progressive aphasia

Features	svPPA	nfvPPA	lvPPA
Spontaneous speech			
Fluency	Normal	Impaired; effortful with false starts and stuttering	Impaired; word-finding difficulties with pauses between words
Grammatical structure	Preserved	Telegraphic with agrammatism	Interruptions may lead to incomplete sentences
Content	Circumlocutory; simplified vocabulary	Preserved	May be circumlocutory
Prosody	Normal	Monotonous	Normal
Paraphasias	Semantic	Phonemic or phonetic	Phonemic and semantic; neologisms
Formal testing			
Speech praxis	Preserved	Impaired	Preserved
Repetition	Preserved	Impaired	Disproportionately impaired for sentences with low-frequency nouns in spoken language
Single-word comprehension	Impaired	Preserved	Preserved
Grammar comprehension	Preserved	Impaired	May be impaired in long sentences
Object knowledge	Impaired	Preserved	Preserved
Reading	Surface dyslexia	Agrammatism; phonemic and phonetic paraphasias	Phonemic errors

Note: lvPPA: logopenic variant of primary progressive aphasia; nfvPPA: nonfluent/agrammatic variant of primary progressive aphasia; svPPA: semantic variant of primary progressive aphasia.

misinterpreted as deficits in complex grammar comprehension (Table 28.2) (Gorno-Tempini et al., 2008).

While language is the leading and dominant issue, other domains often associated with Alzheimer disease can be affected later on, including calculation, memory (often an amnestic pattern), praxis and visuospatial abilities (Owens et al., 2018). Other than myoclonus, which may be perioral, movement disorders are rare. The presence of parkinsonism appears to segregate more commonly with nfvPPA (Graff-Radford et al., 2012). Asymmetric motor (e.g., dystonia, parkinsonism, myoclonus) and cortical sensory findings (e.g., apraxia, cortical sensory loss) in patients with lvPPA would be consistent with the corticobasal syndrome.

Structural imaging in patients with lvPPA reveals atrophy in the temporoparietal junction of the dominant hemisphere resulting in widening of the Sylvian fissure (Gorno-Tempini et al., 2011). Functional neuroimaging studies show a similar pattern of hypometabolism (Gorno-Tempini et al., 2011). CSF biomarkers can be helpful determining if underlying AD pathology is present.

Diagnosis: Logopenic variant of primary progressive aphasia, due to probable Alzheimer disease

Tip: Disrupted output in logopenic speech is due to pauses caused by word-retrieval deficits but normal fluency. On the other hand, nonfluent speech is characterized by effortful, telegraphic speech often associated with false starts, groping, articulatory errors which are features of apraxia of speech. While repetition is affected in both cases, it disproportionately affects long sentences in logopenic speech.

References

Baddeley, A. D. and Hitch, G. J. 2019. The phonological loop as a buffer store: an update. *Cortex* **112** 91–106.

Gorno-Tempini, M. L. et al. 2008. The logopenic/phonological variant of primary progressive aphasia. *Neurology* **71**(16) 1227–1234.

Gorno-Tempini, M. L. et al. 2011. Classification of primary progressive aphasia and its variants. *Neurology* **76**(11) 1006–1014.

Graff-Radford, J., Duffy, J. R., Strand, E. A. and Josephs, K. A. 2012. Parkinsonian motor features distinguish the agrammatic from logopenic variant of primary progressive aphasia. *Parkinsonism Relat Disord* **18**(7) 890–892.

Marshall, C. R. et al. 2018. Primary progressive aphasia: a clinical approach. *J Neurol* **265**(6) 1474–1490.

Owens, T. E. et al. 2018. Patterns of neuropsychological dysfunction and cortical volume changes in logopenic aphasia. *J Alzheimers Dis* **66**(3) 1015–1025.

Rohrer, J. D. et al. 2008. Word-finding difficulty: a clinical analysis of the progressive aphasias. *Brain* **131** (Pt 1) 8–38.

Snowden, J. S. et al. 2007. Cognitive phenotypes in Alzheimer's disease and genetic risk. *Cortex* **43**(7) 835–845.

Wilson, S. M. et al. 2010. Connected speech production in three variants of primary progressive aphasia. *Brain* **133**(Pt 7) 2069–2088.

Case: This 69-year-old right-handed woman presented with 3-year history of progressive memory problems. Her husband described her initial difficulty was recalling recent events along with repeating stories. Within a year, she struggled with reading and with recognizing people, which she attributed to a change in vision. An ophthalmologic evaluation revealed bilateral cataracts, which were surgically corrected. However, her visual abilities continued to decline after surgery. She started having difficulties identifying objects and judging distances, which led her to stop driving. She denied any issues with her memory and attributed all of her problems to her vision, although she could not elaborate further. Her exam was remarkable for a circumlocutory discourse. Her Montreal Cognitive Assessment (MoCA) score was 12/30 due to impairments in trail making, cube copying, clock drawing, naming, serial sevens, phonemic fluency, delayed recall (she could not recall any words freely and recognized only one when multiple choices were given), and orientation to month and date. A recent brain MRI showed generalized atrophy, including bilateral hippocampal atrophy, a pattern suggestive of Alzheimer disease.

With a Tentative Diagnosis of Alzheimer Disease, Is Further Cognitive Testing Necessary?

A cognitive evaluation aims to make three determinations: the underlying pathology, the cognitive domains affected, and the severity of the condition. Identifying the underlying pathology can bring early diagnostic closure, offer a measure of prognosis, and ascertain additional deficits which may have a functional impact. Proper characterization of cognitive deficits should not be overlooked even when the pathologic diagnosis is clear, as they can help the caregivers understand the source of the deficits, guide therapy and assist with decisions regarding living accommodations.

In this case, while her presentation was highly suggestive of Alzheimer disease her deficits went beyond memory impairment, indicating possible visuospatial

dysfunction too. On further bedside evaluation, she exhibited limb ideomotor apraxia and simultanagnosia (Video 29.1). Neuropsychological evaluation revealed severe impairments in memory encoding and visuospatial abilities and moderate deficits in naming, most of which were visual errors rather than paraphasic.

Discussion

Impairments in visual processing are often overlooked as they can be difficult to describe by the patient or may be attributed to deficits in other domains. Therefore, visual processing should be separately evaluated, even if deficits in other cognitive domains have been identified. The current model of cortical visual processing places the primary visual cortex in the striate cortex of the occipital lobe and two divergent processing pathways (Table 29.1) (Goodale and Milner, 1992). Damage to these regions can lead to impaired processing due to direct damage of a key processing region (e.g., simultanagnosia) or disconnection between two regions (e.g., alexia without agraphia) (Mesulam, 1998).

Occipital lesions can lead to impairments in vision, ranging from visual field cuts to cortical blindness (Aldrich et al., 1987). In some cases, while perception of the images is impaired, motion can be perceived, known as Riddoch's phenomenon. In other cases, patients may be unconsciously able to locate objects even if they cannot see them, which is known as blindsight (Barton, 2014). Finally, some patients are unaware of their deficits (i.e., visual anosognosia) and confabulate when asked to describe objects, which is known as Anton syndrome (Aldrich et al., 1987).

The ventral (occipitotemporal) stream, known as the "what" pathway, is involved in processes of recognition (e.g., object, face, color). Disruption of the ventral pathway is associated with visual agnosia, described as the inability to recognize objects through vision while recognition through other modalities is preserved. Visual agnosias can be classified as associative or apperceptive, based on whether the ability to form the accurate visual representation necessary to

---

Video 29.1 The examination demonstrates simultanagnosia when presented with complex images.

Table 29.1 Features of selected syndromes of impaired visual processing

Syndrome	Reported deficit and important distinctions	Evaluation	Localization	Associated findings
Ventral pathway				
Central hemiachromatopsia	Discriminating colors in one visual field	Ishihara plates Farnsworth–Munsell hue test	Contralateral lingual and fusiform gyri	Ipsilateral homonymous superior quadrantanopia
Visual agnosia	Identifying objects and their use through vision; intact identification through other modalities	Object description, naming, use and drawing	Bilateral occipitotemporal	Prosopagnosia
Color anomia[a]	Naming colors (can match and discriminate colors)	Naming colors	Left occipitotemporal	Right hemianopia Alexia without agraphia
Prosopagnosia[a]	Recognizing faces Can identify people by voice, touch, or description	Naming famous people	Right or bilateral fusiform gyri	Visual agnosia
Topographagnosia[a]	Recognizing familiar places and landmarks	Naming famous landmarks	Right medial occipitotemporal	Prosopagnosia
Pure alexia (alexia without agraphia)	Reading Intact abilities to spell but not read what is written	Reading a text Writing	Left occipital lobe and splenium of the corpus callosum Left fusiform gyrus	Right homonymous hemianopia
Dorsal pathway				
Akinetopsia	Perception of continuous motion	Moving images	Bilateral medial superior temporal area	May be unilateral (contralateral lesion)
Asteropsis	Depth perception	Titmus Stereo Fly test	Bilateral occipitoparietal lesions	
Simultanagnosia	Difficulty recognizing detailed objects or scenes Overwhelmed with multiple visual stimuli	Navon letter Arcimboldo paintings Boston cookie theft picture	Bilateral medial occipitoparietal junction, angular gyrus cuneus and intraparietal sulcus.	Optic ataxia Oculomotor apraxia
Optic ataxia	Inaccurate reaching under visual guidance	Reaching objects (impaired) and touching body parts (normal)	Bilateral occipitoparietal.	Simultanagnosia Oculomotor apraxia
Oculomotor apraxia	Reading Searching for objects	Initiation and guidance of saccades and pursuit on command	Bilateral occipitoparietal. Bilateral frontal eye field	Simultanagnosia Optic ataxia
Hemineglect	Identifying the presence of objects in the hemifield	Line bisection Cancellation tasks	Right parietal lobe	Apraxia

[a] Can also be considered a domain-specific agnosia, which can be subclassified in apperceptive and associative.

recognize an object is preserved or not, respectively (Riddoch et al., 2008). This can be evaluated by asking the patient to copy or match the presented object. Visual agnosias can also be domain-specific, affecting recognition of faces (i.e., prosopagnosia) or color (i.e., achromatopsia).

The dorsal (parietal) stream, known as the "where" pathway, processes the visual input in space (Barton, 2014). This type of processing is necessary for perception of depth and motion, and also integration of different visual stimuli into one image. The dorsal stream also plays a role in visual attention, which is relevant to the previously described functions. Disruption of the dorsal pathway may affect at least one of three visual processing mechanisms (Barton, 2011). The first one is impaired perception of the object in space, which leads to deficits like optic ataxia and akinetopsia. The second one is impaired ability to integrate the different visualized elements into one image, simultanagnosia (Beh et al., 2015). Finally, deficits in sensory attention are often seen with right parietal damage, resulting in lack of awareness of sensory stimuli, including visual, in the left hemispace (Hier et al., 1983). Visual neglect may be the more striking finding and should be differentiated from hemianopsia.

Patients with cognitive impairment in which deficits in visual processing are identified should be referred to a low vision specialist, who can help with the use of assisting devices, in addition to physical and occupational therapists, who can provide training on how to adapt to the visual processing deficits. Finally, living arrangements may need to change in order to avoid accidents and mistaking objects (see chapter 10).

Diagnosis: Possible Alzheimer disease with severe memory and visuospatial impairment

Tip: Deficits of visual processing may be overlooked or attributed to deficits in other domains in the absence of a comprehensive assessment of cognitive domains.

References

Aldrich, M. S., Alessi, A. G., Beck, R. W. and Gilman, S. 1987. Cortical blindness: etiology, diagnosis, and prognosis. *Ann Neurol* **21**(2) 149–158.

Barton, J. J. 2011. Disorder of higher visual function. *Curr Opin Neurol* **24**(1) 1–5.

Barton, J. J. 2014. Higher cortical visual deficits. *Continuum* **20**(4) 922–941.

Beh, S. C. et al. 2015. Hiding in plain sight: a closer look at posterior cortical atrophy. *Pract Neurol* **15**(1) 5–13.

Goodale, M. A. and Milner, A. D. 1992. Separate visual pathways for perception and action. *Trends Neurosci* **15**(1) 20–25.

Hier, D. B., Mondlock, J. and Caplan, L. R. 1983. Behavioral abnormalities after right hemisphere stroke. *Neurology* **33**(3) 337–344.

Mesulam, M. M. 1998. From sensation to cognition. *Brain* **121**(6) 1013–1052.

Riddoch, M. J. et al. 2008. A tale of two agnosias: distinctions between form and integrative agnosia. *Cogn Neuropsychol* **25**(1) 56–92.

Case: This 52-year-old left-handed woman with a 10-year history of multiple sclerosis (MS) developed fluctuating affect over the last year. Her children described she cried or laughed inappropriately, without a clear trigger. These episodes lasted less than 10 minutes. Even in the occasions where there was an emotion-triggering event, the response (crying or laughing) was disproportionate and contrary to the expectations (i.e., laughing at something sad). These episodes of laughter and crying were beyond her control and lasted a couple of minutes. Although the patient endorsed being frustrated about these episodes, and endorsed fatigue and slowness in her thinking, she denied persistence in feeling sad, lacking interests or thinking about death. On exam, she exhibited a spastic-ataxic speech and generalized ataxia with spasticity in her upper extremities. Her Beck Depression Inventory (BDI) score was 11, meeting threshold for mild mood disturbance (discouraged about the future, not enjoying things, feeling disappointed about her life, crying more, being more irritable, taking longer to make decisions, being concerned about her looks, needing extra effort to do things, difficulties sleeping, and being worried about her health).

Are the Behaviors within the Spectrum of Depression?

While a number of symptoms she reports are included in the DSM-5 diagnostic criteria for major depressive episode, some of them (e.g., cognitive and motor slowing, fatigue) can also be associated with MS. Indeed, the reported severity of her depressive symptoms seem to be within the expected range of cognitive and motor limitations caused by MS. The presence of abrupt, unexpected laughter and crying represented emotional lability, and the incongruence with the underlying affect and her inability to control them is consistent with pseudobulbar affect (PBA) rather than depression.

Discussion

Disorders of emotion are common in neurodegenerative diseases. Separating the emotional impact of the diagnosis of and disability associated with having a neurodegenerative disease from a pathologic process directly affecting emotional processing is a major clinical challenge. Disorders of emotion can be divided into those where mood disturbances predominate and those where affect is the predominant feature (Arciniegas, 2005). Mood and affect can be defined by two different parameters: duration and physical expression of the emotional state. Based on the duration of the emotional state, mood is defined as the individual's emotional baseline, stable over weeks or months, and affect as an emotional state of short duration, usually minutes to hours. On the other hand, considering the expression of the emotional state, mood is defined as what is the individual's internal emotional state, while affect is the emotional state manifested externally and observed by others (e.g., crying).

PBA is a syndrome of affect dysregulation characterized by typically brief episodes of often intense uncontrollable crying or laughing triggered by trivial stimuli. The frequency of these episodes can vary from occasional to multiple a day. The emergence of pseudobulbar affect is thought to be related to the disruption of cortico-pontine-cerebellar fibers involved in emotional regulation (Parvizi et al., 2009). PBA is not disease-specific but can be present in any condition that disrupts this circuit, including stroke, amyotrophic lateral sclerosis, multiple sclerosis, trauma, and neurodegenerative parkinsonism, more often progressive supranuclear palsy than Parkinson disease (Brooks et al., 2013; Phuong et al., 2009). The emotions expressed are not reflecting underlying feelings and can lead to embarrassment in social situations and impair quality of life, as well as confusion among family members and clinicians regarding the patient's prevalent mood (Colamonico et al., 2012).

PBA is different from mood disorders in terms of duration and congruency with the patient's subjective mood. The minutes-long duration of mood-incongruent PBA should be differentiated from the weeks-long duration of mood-congruent depression. Interestingly, it has been suggested that crying may be reduced in depression and patients may not be able to cry when appropriate (Rottenberg et al., 2008). The presence of other symptoms of depression, including anhedonia, feelings of hopelessness and helplessness, suicide or death ideation, and guilt, are not expected in PBA.

However, it is important to underscore that the presence of depression does not exclude PBA, as they often coexist (Sauve, 2016).

When PBA is expressed as pathological laughter in MS it can be interpreted as euphoria, leading to a misdiagnosis of bipolar disorder. In this case, the lack of pressured speech, grandiosity, flight of ideas, or decreased need for sleep help in the differentiation with mania (Sauve, 2016). Given the brief and sometimes stereotypical nature of PBA, these episodes may also suggest gelastic seizures (such as those associated with hypothalamic hamartomas) or dacrystic seizures associated with temporal lobe epilepsy (Blumberg et al., 2012; Tran et al., 2014). Finally, damage to the frontal lobe, including frontotemporal dementia, can occasionally lead to the syndrome of *Witzelsucht*, in which patients experience increased and inappropriate jocularity, with a tendency to make puns or tell inappropriate jokes (Granadillo and Mendez, 2016).

Clinical criteria for PBA have been proposed, focused on the episodic and involuntary nature of the manifestations along with their incongruency with the underlying mood (Table 30.1) (Miller et al., 2011). A number of scales exist to measure the severity of the symptoms, including the Center for Neurological-Study Lability Scale (CNS-LS) and Pathological Laughing and Crying Scale (PLACS) (Moore et al., 1997; Work et al., 2011). Treatment of PBA should begin by addressing the underlying condition associated with it. Unfortunately, disease-specific treatments for the disorders in which PBA occurs are not known to reduce the severity or frequency of PBA. The combination of dextromethorphan and quinidine is an FDA-approved medication for the treatment of PBA in MS or ALS (Rosen, 2008). In addition, tricyclic antidepressants (e.g., amitriptyline and nortriptyline) and selective serotonin reuptake inhibitors (e.g., citalopram, fluoxetine, and sertraline) have been shown to be effective in small trials for stroke- and MS-associated PBA (Miller et al., 2011).

Diagnosis: Pseudobulbar affect in multiple sclerosis

Tip: Mood and affect represent two different dimensions of emotional processing. Pseudobulbar affect represents a disorder of affect regulation in which the emotional manifestations are incongruent with the individual's internal emotional state.

Table 30.1 Criteria for pseudobulbar affect

Essential criteria
- Episodes of involuntary or exaggerated emotional expression, including episodes of laughing, crying, or related emotional behaviors
  - Episodes represent a change in the patient's usual emotional reactivity, are exaggerated or incongruent with the patient's subjective emotional state and are independent from or disproportionate from the eliciting stimulus.
  - Episodes cause significant distress or impairment in social or occupational functioning.
  - No other neurologic or psychiatric disorder or substance effect can explain the episodes.

Supportive criteria
- Accompanying autonomic changes (e.g., flushing of face) and pseudobulbar signs (e.g., increased jaw jerk, exaggerated gag reflex, tongue weakness, dysarthria and dysphagia)
- Proneness to anger

Source: Adapted from Miller et al. (2011).

References

Arciniegas, D. B. 2005. A clinical overview of pseudobulbar affect. *Am J Geriatr Pharmacother* 3 4–8.

Blumberg, J. et al. 2012. Dacrystic seizures: demographic, semiologic, and etiologic insights from a multicenter study in long-term video-EEG monitoring units. *Epilepsia* 53(10) 1810–1819.

Brooks, B. R. et al. 2013. PRISM: a novel research tool to assess the prevalence of pseudobulbar affect symptoms across neurological conditions. *PLoS One* 8(8) e72232.

Colamonico, J., Formella, A. and Bradley, W. 2012. Pseudobulbar affect: burden of illness in the USA. *Adv Ther* 29(9) 775–798.

Granadillo, E. D. and Mendez, M. F. 2016. Pathological joking or Witzelsucht revisited. *J Neuropsychiatry Clin Neurosci* 28(3) 162–167.

Miller, A., Pratt, H. and Schiffer, R. B. 2011. Pseudobulbar affect: the spectrum of clinical presentations, etiologies and treatments. *Expert Rev Neurother* 11(7) 1077–1088.

Moore, S. R. et al. 1997. A self report measure of affective lability. *J Neurol Neurosurg Psychiatry* 63(1) 89–93.

Parvizi, J. et al. 2009. Neuroanatomy of pathological laughing and crying: a report of the American Neuropsychiatric Association Committee on Research. *J Neuropsychiatry Clin Neurosci* 21(1) 75–87.

Phuong, L. et al. 2009. Involuntary emotional expression disorder (IEED) in Parkinson's disease. *Parkinsonism and Related Disord* 15(7) 511–515.

Rosen, H. 2008. Dextromethorphan/quinidine sulfate for pseudobulbar affect. *Drugs Today* **44**(9) 661–668.

Rottenberg, J., Cevaal, A. and Vingerhoets, A. J. 2008. Do mood disorders alter crying? A pilot investigation. *Depress Anxiety* **25**(5) E9–15.

Sauve, W. M. 2016. Recognizing and treating pseudobulbar affect. *CNS Spectr* **21**(S1) 34–44.

Tran, T. P. et al. 2014. Different localizations underlying cortical gelastic epilepsy: case series and review of literature. *Epilepsy Behav* **35** 34–41.

Work, S. S., Colamonico, J. A., Bradley, W. G. and Kaye, R. E. 2011. Pseudobulbar affect: an under-recognized and under-treated neurological disorder. *Adv Ther* **28**(7) 586–601.

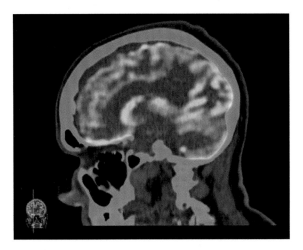

1 FDG-PET scan. This sagittal view shows right orbitofrontal hypometabolism. A black and white version of this figure will appear in some formats.

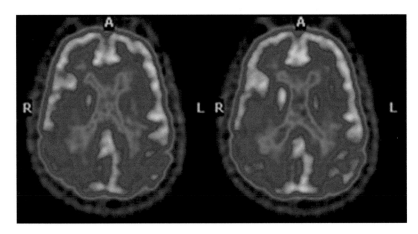

2 FDG-PET in this patient. Note the biparietal and occipital hypometabolism, which is slightly worse on the right. A black and white version of this figure will appear in some formats.

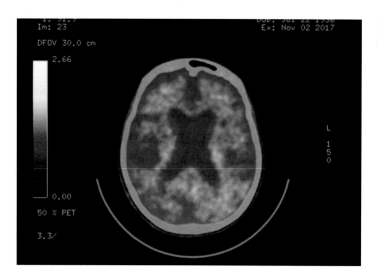

3 Axial cut of Flobetapir amyloid scan showing amyloid deposition. A black and white version of this figure will appear in some formats.

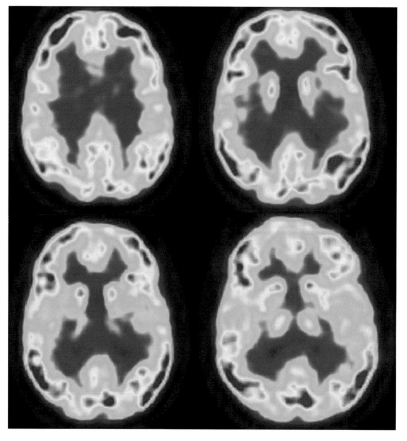

4 Brain FDG-PET in this patient. Note the hypometabolism in the parietal and anterior temporal lobes, bilaterally, with normal activity noted in the basal ganglia and remainder of the brain parenchyma. A black and white version of this figure will appear in some formats.

31 | Does a Positive Amyloid Scan Always Mean Alzheimer Disease?

Case: This 72-year-old left-handed man presented with a 3-year history of cognitive and behavioral decline. His wife first noticed that he was slower to respond and make decisions. He daydreamed and often lost his focus, requiring that comments be repeated. Worsening of symptoms prompted a neurological evaluation within a year of symptom onset. The neurological exam was reported as unremarkable. The score on the Montreal Cognitive Assessment (MoCA) was 24/30 due to impairments in trail making, cube and clock drawings, phonemic fluency, and delayed recall (he recalled three words freely and recognized the other two when multiple choices were given). Brain MRI showed diffuse atrophy. Florbetapir beta-amyloid PET scan was positive by clinical read (Figure 31.1). This led to a diagnosis of Alzheimer disease. He was started on donepezil 5 mg and increased up to 10 mg, which improved his attention for approximately six months. Subsequently, his family reported episodic confusion and inattention with frequent staring spells. This was initially attributed to low blood pressure but discontinuation of antihypertensives did not provide benefit. In addition, he became intermittently confused, particularly at night, and he would be often found talking to imaginary people in the room. During sleep, his wife noticed worsening of his nightmares with frequent thrashing. He remained independent in his activities of daily living, but his family grew increasingly concerned.

On exam, he was alert and fully oriented. He exhibited hypomimia and his speech was soft. Mild cogwheel rigidity was present in both arms. He displayed subtle symmetric slowness with no decrement in amplitude or speed with sequential tapping. His gait was somewhat slow with preserved arm swing and postural reflexes.

Should We Attribute His Decline to the Progression of Alzheimer Disease?

Considering Alzheimer disease (AD) entails the presence of two pathologies (i.e., beta-amyloid and paired helical filament tau); the sole presence of beta-amyloid does not fulfill the criteria to diagnose AD,

the presence of phosphorylated tau (p-tau) is also required. This latter can be ascertained by CSF biomarkers or tau PET imaging.

Despite the presence of beta-amyloid, some elements in his presentation suggested an alternative diagnosis of dementia with Lewy bodies (DLB). First, the episodes initially labeled as daydreaming, and later inattention and confusion, likely represented cognitive fluctuations. Second, hallucinations (visual or auditory) are the most likely reason for the episodes during which he was talking to imaginary people in the room. Moreover, the report of worsening nightmares with frequent thrashing raises the concern of dream enactment behavior (i.e., REM sleep behavior disorder, or RBD), which occur in approximately 75 percent of synucleinopathies long-term. Finally, the relative preservation of memory in the context of impaired executive and visuospatial function suggests a cognitive profile more consistent with early DLB rather than early Alzheimer disease (AD).

On further questioning the patient endorsed seeing people in the room at night. He described them as well-defined men and women he had never met before. He denied having anosmia or constipation. He also reported feeling sad at times, but not anxious.

How Can the Presence of Amyloid, Suggestive of Alzheimer Disease, Be Explained?

Although Lewy bodies (LB) are considered the hallmark of DLB, concurrent AD pathology, particularly beta-amyloid deposition, is observed in approximately two-thirds of autopsies of patients with DLB (Irwin et al., 2017). This should be considered when interpreting the presence of beta-amyloid with either CSF or amyloid PET scan. While helpful to establish the presence of beta-amyloid and AD pathology, the ascertainment of these biomarkers does not inform us about the presence or absence of concurrent pathologies or distinguish between AD, DLB, and Parkinson disease dementia (PDD).

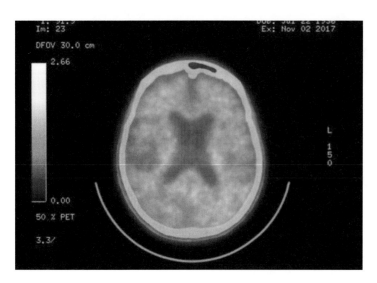

Figure 31.1 Axial cut of Flobetapir amyloid scan showing amyloid deposition. For the colour version, please refer to the plate section.

Discussion

AD and DLB are the most frequent neurodegenerative dementias in the elderly. Although AD and DLB are considered distinct clinical entities, AD pathology often coexists with LB pathology. In fact, data from 213 patients with autopsy-confirmed Lewy body disease show the co-occurrence of beta-amyloid and tau pathologies reach nearly 80 percent, which challenges the notion of "comorbidity" and suggests that there may be common, or synergistic, biological processes leading to pathologies we currently classify as separate (Irwin et al., 2017). This emphasizes the challenge of interpreting imaging and CSF biomarkers. Therefore, we continue to rely on clinical features along with neurobiological markers to help distinguish between AD, DLB, and other dementing disorders (Table 31.1).

The presence of cognitive changes is a core feature in for both AD and DLB. Typical AD presents with a primarily amnestic cognitive syndrome with deficits in memory encoding. DLB on the other hand, usually presents with deficits in executive function and visuospatial abilities initially. Memory impairment usually appears later in DLB, and is usually associated with impaired attention or retrieval, rather than impaired encoding. In addition, the early presence of cognitive fluctuations, reported as decreased level of attention, incoherent speech, or "being in a daze," is a core feature of DLB (McKeith et al., 2017). Fluctuations may be present in more advanced stages of other neurodegenerative disorders, although they are less frequent (Escandon et al., 2010).

Neuropsychiatric features of depression and anxiety are common in both pathologies. The presence of recurrent well-formed visual hallucinations should raise the concern for DLB. Delusions of theft and infidelity may be seen in both syndromes. However, misidentification syndromes, like Capgras (the belief that a familiar person has been replaced by an impostor), are more often seen in the context of DLB (Josephs, 2007).

Parkinsonism is another core feature of DLB, present in up to 85 percent of patients (Fujishiro et al., 2008). However, about a third of patients with AD present parkinsonian features as well, although these typically occur at later stages (Horvath et al., 2014). The absence of parkinsonism in the context of other DLB features is one of the main reasons for missing the diagnosis of DLB.

A history of RBD, suggested by the presence of dream enactment behaviors, is another core diagnostic feature of DLB and is rarely present in nonsynucleinopathies such as AD (McKeith et al., 2017). RBD symptoms may be present up to 50 years before the onset of cognitive or motor symptoms, becoming less frequent or severe as the disease progresses (Claassen et al., 2010; Postuma et al., 2009). Other clinical features supportive of DLB include antipsychotic sensitivity and autonomic abnormalities, including orthostatic hypotension, anosmia, and constipation (McKeith et al., 2017).

Finally, despite the caveats mentioned above, ancillary studies can be helpful in the differential

Table 31.1 Diagnostic criteria for dementia with Lewy bodies

Core clinical features (usually present early)
- Fluctuating cognition with pronounced variations in attention and alertness
- Recurrent visual hallucinations that are typically well formed and detailed
- REM sleep behavior disorder, which may precede cognitive decline
- One or more spontaneous cardinal features of parkinsonism: these are bradykinesia (defined as slowness of movement and decrement in amplitude or speed), rest tremor, or rigidity[a]

Supportive clinical features
- Severe sensitivity to antipsychotic agents
- Postural instability, repeated falls
- Syncope or other transient episodes of unresponsiveness (may be difficult to differentiate from cognitive fluctuation)
- Severe autonomic dysfunction (e.g., constipation, orthostatic hypotension, urinary incontinence)
- Hypersomnia
- Hyposmia
- Hallucinations in other modalities
- Systematized delusions
- Apathy
- Anxiety
- Depression

Indicative biomarkers
- Reduced dopamine transporter uptake in basal ganglia demonstrated by SPECT or PET
- Abnormal (low uptake) [123]iodine-MIBG myocardial scintigraphy
- Polysomnographic confirmation of REM sleep without atonia

Supportive biomarkers
- Relative preservation of medial temporal lobe structures on CT/MRI scan
- Generalized low uptake on SPECT/PET perfusion/metabolism scan with reduced occipital activity ± the cingulate island sign on FDG-PET imaging
- Prominent posterior slow-wave activity on EEG with periodic fluctuations in the pre-alpha/theta range

Probable DLB can be diagnosed if
- Two or more core clinical features of DLB are present, with or without the presence of indicative biomarkers, OR
- Only one core clinical feature is present, but with one or more indicative biomarkers

Possible DLB can be diagnosed if
- Only one core clinical feature of DLB is present, with no indicative biomarker evidence, OR
- One or more indicative biomarkers is present but there are no core clinical features

[a] Parkinsonism mandates the presence of bradykinesia, defined as slowness of movement and decrement in amplitude or speed as movements are continued, along with either resting tremor or rigidity (Postuma et al., 2015).
Source: Adapted from McKeith et al. (2017).

assessment of AD and DLB (Table 31.2). Sparing of the hippocampus on brain MRI (Figure 31.2) and hypometabolism of the occipital cortex with sparing of the posterior cingulate cortex, the latter the so-called cingulate island sign, suggest DLB (McKeith et al., 2017). Nigrostriatal dopamine transporter and postganglionic sympathetic cardiac innervation abnormalities are also characteristic of DLB (Yousaf et al., 2018). EEG abnormalities, specifically pre-alpha-dominant frequency, either stable or inter-mixed with alpha/theta/delta activities in a pseudoperiodic pattern, are also suggestive of DLB rather than AD (Bonanni et al., 2008).

Diagnosis: Dementia with Lewy bodies with positive amyloid scan

Tip: The presence of early nonamnestic cognitive deficits, cognitive fluctuations, hallucinations, and parkinsonism should favor the diagnosis of DLB over AD, regardless of positive amyloid biomarkers (e.g., PET or CSF).

References

Bonanni, L. et al. 2008. EEG comparisons in early Alzheimer's disease, dementia with Lewy bodies and Parkinson's disease with dementia patients with a 2-year follow-up. *Brain* **131**(Pt 3) 690–705.

Claassen, D. O. et al. 2010. REM sleep behavior disorder preceding other aspects of synucleinopathies by up to half a century. *Neurology* **75**(6) 494–499.

Table 31.2 Selected imaging findings in the differentiation between DLB and AD

	Dementia with Lewy bodies	Alzheimer disease
MRI	Mild cortical atrophy with relative sparing of MTL and hippocampus	Atrophy of MTL and hippocampus
Glucose PET	Occipital hypometabolism Preservation of posterior cingulate cortex	Temporo-parietal and posterior cingulate hypometabolism
Amyloid PET	Positive amyloid deposition (frequent)	Positive amyloid deposition (always)
Tau PET	Absent – slightly abnormal uptake in some cases in temporoparietal and occipital cortex	Positive tau deposition (always)
DaTScan	Reduced striatal uptake	Normal
MIBG myocardial scintigraphy	Reduced uptake	Normal

Note: DaTScan: dopamine transporter scan; MTL: medial temporal lobe; PET: positron emission tomography; MIBG: metaiodobenzylguanidine.

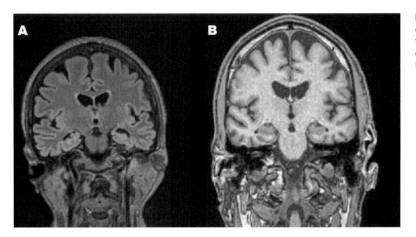

Figure 31.2 FLAIR coronal brain MRI distinguishing AD from DLB. The mesial temporal lobe is (A) atrophic in Alzheimer disease but (B) preserved in dementia with Lewy bodies.

Escandon, A., Al-Hammadi, N. and Galvin, J. E. 2010. Effect of cognitive fluctuation on neuropsychological performance in aging and dementia. *Neurology* **74**(3) 210–217.

Fujishiro, H. et al. 2008. Validation of the neuropathologic criteria of the third consortium for dementia with Lewy bodies for prospectively diagnosed cases. *J Neuropathol Exp Neurol* **67**(7) 649–656.

Horvath, J. et al. 2014. Neuropathology of parkinsonism in patients with pure Alzheimer's disease. *J Alzheimers Dis* **39** (1) 115–120.

Irwin, D. J. et al. 2017. Neuropathological and genetic correlates of survival and dementia onset in synucleinopathies: a retrospective analysis. *Lancet Neurol* **16** (1) 55–65.

Josephs, K. A. 2007. Capgras syndrome and its relationship to neurodegenerative disease. *Arch Neurol* **64**(12) 1762–1766.

McKeith, I. G. et al. 2017. Diagnosis and management of dementia with Lewy bodies: fourth consensus report of the DLB Consortium. *Neurology* **89**(1) 88–100.

Postuma, R. B. et al. 2015. MDS clinical diagnostic criteria for Parkinson's disease. *Mov Disord* **30**(12) 1591–1601.

Postuma, R. B., Gagnon, J. F., Vendette, M. and Montplaisir, J. Y. 2009. Idiopathic REM sleep behavior disorder in the transition to degenerative disease. *Mov Disord* **24**(15) 2225–2232.

Yousaf, T., Dervenoulas, G., Valkimadi, P. E. and Politis, M. 2018. Neuroimaging in Lewy body dementia. *J Neurol* **266** (1) 1–26.

Herpes Encephalitis Recurrence?

Case: This 52-year-old man presented to the emergency room with aggressive behavior and emotional lability progressing over the previous three days. He had completed a three-week course of acyclovir for the treatment of herpes simplex encephalitis (HSE) two weeks prior. Other than residual mild memory difficulties, he was fully functional until his more recent behavioral changes. He was afebrile and his vitals were within normal limits. He was irritable and his attention fluctuated. His exam otherwise unremarkable. MRI of the brain with and without contrast was unremarkable. Laboratory results were significant only for mildly increased CSF protein (100 mg/dl normal range: 15–45 mg/dl). Given the concern of HSE relapse, he was placed on acyclovir again.

Is There Anything Else We Should Consider?

While a recurrence of HSV is possible, his abrupt behavioral decline after appropriate treatment and CSF only remarkable for elevate protein warrants for other possibilities to be considered. The immune response to infectious processes targeting the nervous system can sometimes lead to the development of antibodies targeting normal structures of the nervous system, also known as a parainfectious process. Therefore, evaluation for autoimmune etiologies, like paraneoplastic antibodies, needs to be considered.

A paraneoplastic panel was sent. His condition continued to deteriorate. His CSF HSV PCR came back negative. NMDA-R antibodies were found to be elevated in serum and CSF. He was started on a five-day course of corticosteroids and his condition improved significantly, returning to baseline after three days treatment.

Discussion

HSE typically follows a monophasic course. However, relapse of symptoms after treatment has been reported in up to 12 percent of patients (Skoldenberg et al., 2006). In a subgroup of these patients, even though HSV is not detected in the CSF, antibodies targeting the neuronal surface are present, suggesting a postinfectious autoimmune process (Armangue et al., 2015). N-methyl-D-aspartate receptor (NMDA-R) antibodies are most commonly detected across all age groups (Armangue et al., 2015). Relapses associated with NMDA-R antibodies occur between 4 and 6 weeks after initial HSV infection (Galli et al., 2017). While children tend to manifest choreoathetosis and encephalopathy, adults typically present with changes in behavior and personality (Galli et al., 2017). MRI with gad may show diffuse confluent leukoencephalopathy with contrast enhancement, which differs from the asymmetric necrotic pattern with evidence of hemorrhage seen in HSE (Armangue et al., 2015). Immunosuppression with either corticosteroids, intravenous immunoglobulin, or plasmapheresis provides significant benefit, with most patients returning to their baseline (Armangue et al., 2015).

Diagnosis: Post-HSV anti-NMDA-R encephalitis

Tip: In the context of possible HSE recurrence, always consider autoimmune etiologies, particularly anti-NMDA-R encephalitis.

References

Armangue, T. et al. 2015. Autoimmune post-herpes simplex encephalitis of adults and teenagers. *Neurology* **85**(20) 1736–1743.

Galli, J., Clardy, S. L. and Piquet, A. L. 2017. NMDAR encephalitis following herpes simplex virus encephalitis. *Curr Infect Dis Rep* **19**(1) 1.

Skoldenberg, B. et al. 2006. Incidence and pathogenesis of clinical relapse after herpes simplex encephalitis in adults. *J Neurol* **253**(2) 163–170.

Case: This 72-year-old left-handed woman presented with a 2-year history of worsening cognitive slowness. Her family first noticed she had difficulties multitasking and was slower to respond. She progressively became forgetful and exhibited episodes, some characterized unintelligible speech, while in other she appeared to be in a daze. Her gait slowed down in the last year and she now walked with a stooped posture, dragging her feet. In addition, her family endorsed anosmia and dream enactment behavior during the review of systems. She had been evaluated for a possible autoimmune/paraneoplastic encephalopathy due to the relatively rapid progression of his symptoms. He was found to have elevated titers of voltage-gate potassium channel complex (VGKCC) antibodies (0.08 nmol/L; normal < 0.02). Leucine-rich glioma inactivated 1 (LGI1) and contactin-associated protein-like 2 (CASPR2) were negative. Given this finding, he underwent a five-day course of intravenous immunoglobulin (IVIg), without subjective or objective (i.e., cognitive testing) improvement.

On exam, she exhibited a symmetric tremorless parkinsonism with hypomimia and hypophonia. Her posture was slightly stooped, and her gait was shuffling. On cognitive evaluation, she exhibited deficits in working memory, processing speed, visuospatial abilities as well as impairments in free recall which improved with cueing, suggesting a retrieval deficit. Her brain MRI was unremarkable.

Should We Proceed with More Aggressive Immunotherapy?

The expansion of the field of neuroimmunology has made antibody testing more accessible, often in the form of panels of antibodies. This may lead to the detection of antibodies which were not considered in the differential diagnosis. Finding antibodies suggestive of autoimmune encephalitis may distract from the findings of a thorough clinical evaluation and lead to unnecessary treatments.

In this case, her symptoms and course of decline were not consistent with limbic encephalitis, but rather with dementia with Lewy bodies (DLB), particularly when considering the presence of anosmia and dream enactment behaviors. Moreover, although

VGKCC antibodies were present, LGI1 and CASPR2 were not, raising the concern of the pathogenic nature of the antibodies found (van Sonderen et al., 2017). Finally, although parkinsonian syndrome have been associated with autoimmune causes (e.g., anti-Ma, anti-IgLON5), there is no clear association between VGKCC and DLB (Dalmau et al., 2004; Gaig et al., 2017). Therefore, this finding should be considered incidental. Therefore, the patient should not undergo further immunotherapy.

Discussion

Autoimmune encephalitis (AE) subacutely affect the level of alertness, behavior, or memory encoding. Ancillary studies (e.g., CSF and MRI) may suggest an inflammatory process. Pleocytosis, oligoclonal bands, or elevated CSF IgG index may be present in CSF. T2-FLAIR brain MRI may show hyperintensities in the medial temporal lobe or in a multifocal cortical and subcortical pattern (Graus et al., 2016). Four distinct syndromes have been recognized (Table 33.1) (Graus et al., 2016). The identification of these syndromes based in their clinical presentation and findings in the ancillary allow the diagnosis of AE before the autoantibody status is known (Graus et al., 2016). However, a substantial number of patients with criteria for AE do not present with a well-defined syndrome and in these cases the detection of specific antibodies establishes the diagnosis. Nevertheless, the presence or absence of antibodies needs to be interpreted in a clinical context. On one hand, the absence of identifiable antibodies in a patient who fulfills the criteria for probable AE or one of the four AE syndromes should not discourage aggressive immunomodulatory treatment. On the other hand, the detection of antibodies in patients not fulfilling these criteria should be interpreted with caution, such as in our case.

VGKCC antibodies targeting LGI1 or CASPR2 subunits are considered pathogenic and are associated with distinct syndromes (See Case 17). About half of patients tested with VGKCC antibodies do not have LGI1 or CASPR2 antibodies (van Sonderen et al., 2017). Most of these cases are associated with a plethora of unrelated symptoms or syndromes of unlikely autoimmune etiology, ranging from pain to

Table 33.1 Clinical and ancillary features of main autoimmune encephalitis syndromes

Syndrome	Limbic encephalitis	Anti-NMDA receptor-antibody encephalitis	Acute disseminated encephalomyelitis	Bickerstaff brainstem encephalitis
Onset	< 3 months	< 4 weeks	*Acute, monophasic* Preceded by flu-like symptoms	<4 weeks Preceded by an infectious event
Cognitive and behavioral features	Anterograde amnesia Changes in personality	Psychosis Speech changes (pressured speech, mutism)	Decreased level of alertness	Decreased level of alertness
Motor features	Seizures *Faciobrachial dystonic seizures (LGI-1)*	Seizures *Oral dyskinesia* *Catatonia*	Ataxia Paresis Myelopathy Cranial neuropathies	*Ataxia* *Bilateral external ophthalmoplegia* Bilateral facial palsy
Other findings	*Hyponatremia (LGI-1)* *Supranuclear gaze palsy (Ma2 and IgLON5)* *Narcolepsy-cataplexy (Ma2)*	Dysautonomia Central hypoventilation	Optic neuropathy	None
Brain MRI	*Bilateral FLAIR hyperintensities in the medial temporal lobe*	Nonspecific FLAIR hyperintensities affecting brain and brainstem; may be normal	*Multiple large (> 2 cm) white matter FLAIR hyperintensities in brain, brainstem, cerebellum, or spinal cord*	Brainstem T2 hyperintensity; may be normal
CSF	Normal/pleocytosis	Normal/pleocytosis	Normal/pleocytosis	Normal/pleocytosis
EEG	Temporal epileptiform activity	Diffuse slowing Epileptiform activity *Delta brush*	Diffuse slowing	Normal
Associated antibodies	VGKCC (LGI-1 or CASPR2) Hu Ma2 AMPA GABAb	GluN1 subunit of NMDA receptor	MOG (transient in children)	GQ1b

Note: Distinct features of these selected syndromes are written in italics. AMPA: α-amino-3-hydroxy-5-methyl-4-isoxazolepropionic acid receptor; CASPR2: contactin-associated protein-like 2; GABAB: gamma-aminobutyric acid receptor b; GQ1B: ganglioside gq1b; MOG: myelin oligodendrocyte glycoprotein; LGI-1: leucine-rich glioma inactivated 1; NMDA: N-methyl-D-aspartate receptor; VGKCC: voltage-gated potassium channel complex.

Asperger syndrome (van Sonderen et al., 2017). Moreover, the VGKCC titer alone is not useful to discriminate between patients with and without an autoimmune pathogenic process or disease severity (Jammoul et al., 2016; van Sonderen et al., 2016). Therefore, VGKCC antibody positivity in the absence of reflex antibodies to LGI1 and CASPR2 is not a clear marker for pathogenic autoimmunity and does not have a clear diagnostic value unless placed in the appropriate clinical context. Finally, LGI1 and CASPR2 antibodies may be present in the absence of VGKC antibodies (van Sonderen et al., 2017). Hence, in the appropriate context (e.g., limbic encephalitis presenting with faciobrachial dystonic seizures) LGI1 and CASPR2 should be investigated even in the absence of VGKCC antibodies.

Diagnosis: Dementia with Lewy bodies with spurious VGKC elevation

Tip: Serum antibodies need to be interpreted in the appropriate clinical context. The pathologic nature of VGKCC antibodies in the absence of LGI1 and CASPR2 antibodies should be questioned, particularly if the clinical presentation is not consistent with an autoimmune encephalitis.

References

Dalmau, J. et al. 2004. Clinical analysis of anti-Ma2-associated encephalitis. *Brain* **127**(8) 1831–1844.

Gaig, C. et al. 2017. Clinical manifestations of the anti-IgLON5 disease. *Neurology* **88**(18) 1736–1743.

Graus, F. et al. 2016. A clinical approach to diagnosis of autoimmune encephalitis. *Lancet Neurol* **15**(4) 391–404.

Jammoul, A. et al. 2016. Clinical utility of seropositive voltage-gated potassium channel-complex antibody. *Neurol Clin Pract* **6**(5) 409–418.

van Sonderen, A. et al. 2016. The relevance of VGKC positivity in the absence of LGI1 and Caspr2 antibodies. *Neurology* **86**(18) 1692–1699.

van Sonderen, A., Petit-Pedrol, M., Dalmau, J. and Titulaer, M. J. 2017. The value of LGI1, Caspr2 and voltage-gated potassium channel antibodies in encephalitis. *Nat Rev Neurol* **13**(5) 290–301.

Case: This 79-year-old left-handed woman presented after six months of progressive cognitive and behavioral changes. She rapidly became forgetful and easily confused, irritable, and had delusional thinking of people trying to harm her emerging over two weeks. Within three months, her language declined to the point where she couldn't follow commands or produce intelligible or coherent speech. Her balance and walking declined, rendering her wheelchair bound. Her prior medication regimen consisted of amlodipine and atorvastatin, with no changes in recent years.

On exam, she was agitated and did not follow commands. Her speech consisted of mostly unintelligible and mumbled verbalizations. She exhibited generalized myoclonus and ataxia.

Prior blood and urine workup for rapidly progressive dementia (Table 34.1) was unremarkable. Cerebrospinal fluid (CSF) analysis done two months earlier showed normal cell count, normal glucose, protein level of 63 mg/dl, and no evidence of protein 14–3–3. RT-QuIC was not done. Brain MRI showed bilateral restricted diffusion in the cerebral cortex as well as in the caudate and putamen (Figure 34.1). EEG showed mild diffuse background slowing and no epileptiform discharges were noted. She was transferred for a diagnostic brain biopsy.

Is a Biopsy an Appropriate Step for Diagnosis in This Case?

In the context of a rapidly progressive dementia, brain biopsy with meningeal tissue may be considered from accessible, noneloquent cortical regions.

Doesn't the Absence of 14–3–3 Protein in CSF and Characteristic EEG Changes Rule Out the Possibility of Prion Disease?

Although traditionally elevated 14–3–3 has been considered a criterion for the diagnosis of sporadic Creutzfeldt–Jakob disease (sCJD) as it represents a nonspecific marker of rapid brain cell death and might be elevated in variety of neurological conditions, including metabolic encephalitis, herpes simplex, hypoxic encephalitis, stroke, and metastatic brain disease (Geschwind et al., 2003). Moreover, the reported sensitivity and specificity for the diagnosis of sCJD has a high variability, ranging from 53 percent to 97 percent and from 40 percent to 100 percent, respectively (Geschwind, 2016). More importantly, the presence of restricted diffusion affecting the cortex and the striatum, along with the increased FLAIR signal affecting the striatum and thalamus, are strongly supportive of sCJD, regardless of a negative 14–3–3.

Repeat CSF examination performed two months later showed high levels of 14–3–3 along with elevated total tau protein and neuron specific enolase.

Discussion

sCJD is the most common prion disease and the archetypal rapidly progressive dementia (RPD). The typical clinical presentation consists of a subacute progressive decline in cognitive, behavioral and motor function, ultimately leading to akinetic mutism and subsequently death within a year of symptom onset. The differential diagnosis of sCJD is extensive and includes several treatable conditions which should always be assessed (Table 34.1). Although pathologic diagnosis remains the gold standard, neuroimaging and CSF analysis can aid the early detection of sCJD. Other features, as EEG abnormalities and the presence of myoclonus and startle are frequently present in sCJD, although at more advanced stages.

Increased DWI signal with corresponding decreased apparent diffusion coefficient (ADC) signal in the thalamus or striatum or cortex (known as cortical ribboning) tend to appear early on brain MRI (Vitali et al., 2011). These findings may represent vacuolization, characteristic of this condition. In addition, increased T2 and FLAIR signal in the striatum may appear later (Meissner et al., 2009). Contrast enhancement is not a feature of sCJD and should raise the suspicion for lymphoma and inflammatory disorders.

CSF analysis in sCJD usually shows no cells and normal glucose, with elevation of protein occurring in about half of cases (Zeidler and Green, 2004). A negative 14–3–3 does not exclude the diagnosis if the

Table 34.1 Selected test to be considered in the assessment of rapidly progressive dementias

Category	Tests	Disorders with abnormalities
Blood tests	• Complete blood cell count with differential • Comprehensive metabolic panel including calcium and magnesium • Liver function tests • Thyroid function • Vitamin B_1 and B_{12} • Rheumatoid screen (ESR, CRP, ANA) • Human immunodeficiency virus • RPR • Medication levels (e.g., lithium, chemotherapy) • Paraneoplastic panel • Lactate and pyruvate • Bismuth levels	• Anemia, infection • Hyponatremia, hypercalcemia • Liver failure • Hypothyroidism • Vitamin deficiency, Wernicke's encephalopathy • Lupus • HIV associated dementia • Syphilis • Toxic levels of medication • Limbic encephalopathy • Mitochondrial disease • Bismuth toxicity
Urine	• Urine analysis with culture • Urine drug screen • Heavy metal screen	• Urinary tract infection • Illegal substance use • Mercury, lead toxicity
CSF	• Cell count with differential, protein, glucose • IgG index, oligoclonal bands • Cytology, flow cytometry • Bacterial, fungal, and acid-fast bacilli stains and culture • Viral PCR • Whipple PCR • NMDA receptor antibodies • 14–3–3, neuron specific enolase • RT-QuIC • Beta-amyloid, total tau, and phosphorylated tau	• Infection, neoplasm • Autoimmune process • Malignancy • Pneumococcus, cryptococcus, tuberculosis • HSV, CMV, EBV • Whipple disease • NMDAR encephalopathy • Markers of rapid neuronal loss • CJD • Alzheimer disease
Others	• Brain MRI with and without contrast • Chest X-ray • EEG	• Stroke, malignancy, infection, demyelinating disorders • Pneumonia • Seizures, status epilepticus

Note: ANA: antinuclear antibody; CJD: Creutzfeldt–Jakob disease; CMV: cytomegalovirus; CRP: C-reactive protein; EBV: Epstein–Barr virus; ESR: eritrosedimentation rate; HSV: herpes simplex virus, NMDAR: N-methyl-D-aspartate receptor; RT-QuIC: real-time quaking-induced conversion.

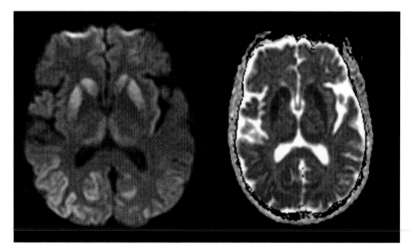

Figure 34.1 Axial diffusion-weighted image (DWI) and apparent diffusion coefficient (ADC) brain MRI. Note the DWI hyperintensities with ADC correlation in the striata, pulvinar, and medial regions of the thalami, along with asymmetric cortical ribboning in the parieto-occipital cortical region.

clinical suspicion is high. Other CSF markers of neuronal damage include elevated total tau and neuron specific enolase, while elevated s100b represents a marker of astrocyte and Schwann cell damage (Zerr et al., 1996). The detection of misfolded (pathogenic) prion protein by real-time quaking-induced conversion (RT-QuIC) has become increasingly available and has shown to be sensitive and specific (91 percent and 98 percent, respectively) for the diagnosis sCJD (McGuire et al., 2012).

The utility of EEG in the assessment of sCJD has been relegated due to availability of more specific tools, such as CSF and MRI. Seizures are rare in sCJD and represent a red flag against the diagnosis of sCJD, instead raising the possibility of infectious, toxic, metabolic and autoimmune encephalopathies. One-per-second sharps or triphasic waves on EEG, known as periodic sharp wave complexes (PSWC), represent a characteristic finding in sCJD (Steinhoff et al., 1996). However, these nonspecific findings are late manifestations and are also expressed in anoxic brain injury and metabolic encephalopathies (Tschampa et al., 2007).

Diagnosis: Creutzfeldt–Jakob disease with a false negative 14–3–3

Tip: This form of rapidly progressive dementia may be overlooked with a negative 14–3–3 but typical brain MRI, and other markers of rapid neuronal loss, particularly abnormal RT-QuIC, can more reliably assist with ascertaining the diagnosis.

References

Geschwind, M. D. 2016. Rapidly progressive dementia. *Continuum* **22**(2) 510–537.

Geschwind, M. D. et al. 2003. Challenging the clinical utility of the 14–3–3 protein for the diagnosis of sporadic Creutzfeldt–Jakob disease. *Arch Neurol* **60**(6) 813–816.

McGuire, L. I. et al. 2012. RT-QuIC analysis of cerebrospinal fluid in sporadic Creutzfeldt–Jakob disease. *Ann Neurol* **72**(2) 278–285.

Meissner, B. et al. 2009. MRI lesion profiles in sporadic Creutzfeldt–Jakob disease. *Neurology* **72**(23) 1994–2001.

Steinhoff, B. J. et al. 1996. Accuracy and reliability of periodic sharp wave complexes in Creutzfeldt–Jakob disease. *Arch Neurol* **53**(2) 162–166.

Tschampa, H. J. et al. 2007. Pattern of cortical changes in sporadic Creutzfeldt–Jakob disease. *AJNR Am J Neuroradiol* **28**(6) 1114–1118.

Vitali, P. et al. 2011. Diffusion-weighted MRI hyperintensity patterns differentiate CJD from other rapid dementias. *Neurology* **76**(20) 1711–1719.

Zeidler, M. and Green, A. 2004. Advances in diagnosing Creutzfeldt–Jakob disease with MRI and CSF 14–3–3 protein analysis. *Neurology* **63**(3) 410–411.

Zerr, I. et al. 1996. Diagnosis of Creutzfeldt–Jakob disease by two-dimensional gel electrophoresis of cerebrospinal fluid. *The Lancet* **348**(9031) 846–849.

You Have Been Diagnosed with Alzheimer Disease; Is That It?

Case: This 51-year-old right-handed woman requested further care for her previously diagnosed Alzheimer disease. Over the previous year, her coworkers observed that she would frequently forget instructions and conversations and increasingly relied on written reminders. She would ask the same question repeatedly and cueing helped inconsistently. Her symptoms had not worsened since. There were no language or visuospatial impairments. Her past medical history included lumpectomy and tamoxifen for breast cancer five years ago, and a 30-year history of alcohol abuse (daily beer and vodka, unknown volume). Indeed, family members reported finding empty bottles of vodka in the garbage. She had no family history of cognitive impairment or other neurologic condition.

Previous work up included a normal blood work, brain MRI with contrast, normal cell count, protein, glucose, and cytology in cerebrospinal fluid, but bilateral temporoparietal hypometabolism on FDG-PET (Figure 35.1). With a presumed diagnosis of Alzheimer disease, she was started on donepezil 5 mg daily.

Cognitive testing demonstrated disorientation in time, impaired working memory, and reduced phonemic and semantic fluency. The CERAD memory task showed poor learning (4 out of 10 words) with intrusions on successive trials. She could only recall 2 words on delayed free recall and 5 out of 10 words with cueing. On motor examination, she showed a symmetric low-amplitude, high-frequency postural tremor.

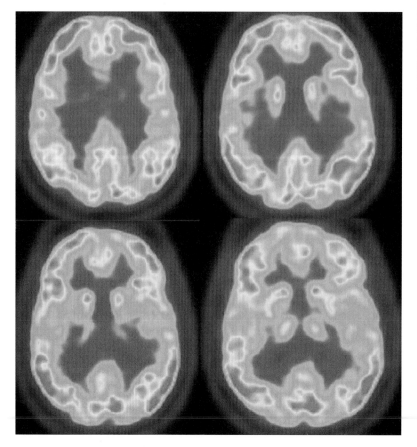

Figure 35.1 Brain FDG-PET in this patient. Note the hypometabolism in the parietal and anterior temporal lobes, bilaterally, with normal activity noted in the basal ganglia and remainder of the brain parenchyma. For the colour version, please refer to the plate section.

Was the Pattern of FDG-PET Hypometabolism Sufficient for the Diagnosis of Alzheimer Disease?

FDG-PET reflects the use of glucose throughout the brain, serving as a surrogate topographic marker of neuronal injury or degeneration based on patterns of hypometabolism. However, it does not serve to support or refute neurodegenerative etiologies in the absence of the appropriate clinical context. Moreover, multiple factors can affect cognition and behavior, and the presence of one does not rule out the existence of others. Although AD cannot be ruled out at this point, the patient's age and the lack of family history of AD should raise the concern for alternative comorbidities. In this case, her history of alcohol abuse should be considered as contributory, even in the presence of AD pathology. In addition, her cancer history and subacute cognitive decline also suggest the possibility of an autoimmune/paraneoplastic etiology. Finally, in every patient who presents with subacute cognitive decline, metabolic, pharmacologic, and sleep-related variables should be investigated as potentially etiologic. Importantly, most of these are also associated with cerebral FDG-PET hypometabolism (Table 35.1) (Berti et al., 2014; Daulatzai, 2017).

In her case, she was found to have a glycated hemoglobin of 6.2 percent, suggestive of prediabetes, and folate levels of 1.7 ng/mL indicative of folate deficiency. As part of her medication regimen she was taking hyoscyamine for abdominal cramps, a medication with known anticholinergic effects. After the acknowledgment of snoring, polysomnography was obtained and demonstrated an apnea/hypopnea index (AHI) of 17, diagnostic of obstructive sleep apnea. Her workup also included a paraneoplastic panel, which was normal, and cerebrospinal measurements of amyloid, total tau and phosphorylated tau, which were also normal, effectively ruling out AD.

Discussion

Biomarkers for AD can be classified in two groups: neurodegenerative and pathophysiologic (Table 35.2). These biomarkers can assist with diagnosis of both symptomatic as well as preclinical neurodegenerative syndromes (Dubois et al., 2016). On one hand, pathophysiological biomarkers determine the presence or absence AD but cannot help ascertaining the areas affected by AD or exclude other concurrent pathologies. In contrast, neurodegenerative markers lack specificity for AD pathology but are helpful in the assessment of its distribution and severity.

Fluorodeoxyglucose positron emission tomography (FDG-PET) measures cerebral glucose metabolism, which is closely associated with synaptic density and function (Rocher et al., 2003). In AD, FDG-PET hypometabolism precedes cognitive impairment by up to 10 years and correlates with the degree of cognitive impairment throughout the course of the disease (Bateman et al., 2012; Engler et al., 2006; Furst et al., 2012; Villemagne et al., 2013). A normal FDG-PET argues against a neurodegenerative disease, but an abnormal one does not confirm it (Perani et al., 2014). FDG-PET has good sensitivity (84–96 percent) but only moderate specificity (73–80 percent) in the diagnosis of AD (Bohnen et al., 2012; Jagust et al., 2007). In classic AD hypometabolism is evidenced first in the medial parietal, including precuneus and posterior cingulate cortex, later spreading to the lateral

Table 35.1 Important comorbidities affecting cognition (FDG-PET hypometabolism-inducing disorders in bold)

	Examples
Metabolic conditions	**Diabetes**, hypothyroidism, **low vitamin B₁₂, low folate**
Vascular	**Hypertension, hypotension**
Infections	Urinary tract infection
Sleep	**Obstructive sleep apnea**
Medications	Medication with anticholinergic burden, **sedatives, opiates**
Substances	**Alcohol, illegal drugs (e.g., cocaine, cannabis, amphetamines)**

Table 35.2 Classification of Alzheimer disease biomarkers

Type	CSF biomarkers	Imaging biomarkers
Neurodegenerative	Elevated total tau	Hippocampal atrophy, temporoparietal hypometabolism by FDG-PET, temporoparietal hypoperfusion by SPECT
Pathophysiologic	**Amyloid:** low Aβ-42 **Tau:** elevated p-tau	**Amyloid:** positive amyloid PET scan **Tau:** positive tau PET scan

temporal lobe and medial frontal regions (Bohnen et al., 2012). These areas are key structures of the large-scale distributed brain network known as the default mode network, which is known to be highly vulnerable to amyloid deposition (Buckner et al., 2005; Raichle, 2015). Alternatively, in atypical variants of AD (e.g., posterior cortical atrophy) the pattern of hypometabolism correlates with the areas of neurodegeneration (e.g., occipital lobe).

Other comorbidities that may disrupt cerebral perfusion and glucose metabolism, which also affect cognition, should be considered. Particular attention should be paid to prediabetes or diabetes, as either may lead to a pattern of temporoparietal hypometabolism similar to the one observed in AD (Roberts et al., 2014). Other conditions associated with FDG-PET hypometabolism include obstructive sleep apnea, hypertension, vitamin B_{12}/folate deficiency, medications (e.g., benzodiazepines, anesthetics), certain substances (e.g., caffeine, alcohol, amphetamines, cocaine), and epileptic seizures (Berti et al., 2014; Daulatzai, 2017).

FDG-PET may be useful in the setting of clinical uncertainty: frontotemporal hypometabolism supports the diagnosis of frontotemporal lobar degeneration while occipital hypometabolism, in addition to temporoparietal with sparing of the cingulate cortex, suggests DLB (Foster et al., 2007; Mosconi et al., 2008). In primary progressive aphasia, asymmetric left frontal, frontoparietal, or temporal hypometabolism can assist in distinguishing among nonfluent, logopenic, and semantic variants, respectively. Also, FDG-PET suggests an increased risk of progression from normal cognition to MCI and ultimately to dementia and may in the future serve as a marker of response to disease-modifying treatments (Johnson et al., 2012; Landau et al., 2010).

Diagnosis: Multifactorial cognitive impairment (likely nonneurodegenerative)

Tip: The clinical context and comorbidities of patients with cognitive impairment should affect the conclusions derived from surrogate markers of neurodegeneration or neuronal dysfunction.

References

Bateman, R. J. et al. 2012. Clinical and biomarker changes in dominantly inherited Alzheimer's disease. *N Engl J Med* **367**(9) 795–804.

Berti, V., Mosconi, L. and Pupi, A. 2014. Brain: normal variations and benign findings in fluorodeoxyglucose-PET/computed tomography imaging. *PET Clin* **9**(2) 129–140.

Bohnen, N. I. et al. 2012. Effectiveness and safety of 18F-FDG PET in the evaluation of dementia: a review of the recent literature. *J Nucl Med* **53**(1) 59–71.

Buckner, R. L. et al. 2005. Molecular, structural, and functional characterization of Alzheimer's disease: evidence for a relationship between default activity, amyloid, and memory. *J Neurosci* **25**(34) 7709–7717.

Daulatzai, M. A. 2017. Cerebral hypoperfusion and glucose hypometabolism: key pathophysiological modulators promote neurodegeneration, cognitive impairment, and Alzheimer's disease. *J Neurosci Res* **95**(4) 943–972.

Dubois, B. et al. 2016. Preclinical Alzheimer's disease: definition, natural history, and diagnostic criteria. *Alzheimers Dement* **12**(3) 292–323.

Engler, H. et al. 2006. Two-year follow-up of amyloid deposition in patients with Alzheimer's disease. *Brain* **129**(Pt 11) 2856–2866.

Foster, N. L. et al. 2007. FDG-PET improves accuracy in distinguishing frontotemporal dementia and Alzheimer's disease. *Brain* **130**(Pt 10) 2616–2635.

Furst, A. J. et al. 2012. Cognition, glucose metabolism and amyloid burden in Alzheimer's disease. *Neurobiol Aging* **33**(2) 215–225.

Jagust, W. et al. 2007. What does fluorodeoxyglucose PET imaging add to a clinical diagnosis of dementia? *Neurology* **69**(9) 871–877.

Johnson, K. A., Fox, N. C., Sperling, R. A. and Klunk, W. E. 2012. Brain imaging in Alzheimer disease. *Cold Spring Harb Perspect Med* **2**(4) a006213.

Landau, S. M. et al. 2010. Comparing predictors of conversion and decline in mild cognitive impairment. *Neurology* **75**(3) 230–238.

Mosconi, L. et al. 2008. Multicenter standardized 18F-FDG PET diagnosis of mild cognitive impairment, Alzheimer's disease, and other dementias. *J Nucl Med* **49**(3) 390–398.

Perani, D. et al. 2014. Validation of an optimized SPM procedure for FDG-PET in dementia diagnosis in a clinical setting. *Neuroimage Clin* **6** 445–454.

Raichle, M. E. 2015. The brain's default mode network. *Annu Rev Neurosci* **38** 433–447.

Roberts, R. O. et al. 2014. Diabetes and elevated hemoglobin A1c levels are associated with brain hypometabolism but not amyloid accumulation. *J Nucl Med* **55**(5) 759–764.

Rocher, A. B. et al. 2003. Resting-state brain glucose utilization as measured by PET is directly related to regional synaptophysin levels: a study in baboons. *Neuroimage* **20**(3) 1894–1898.

Villemagne, V. L. et al. 2013. Amyloid beta deposition, neurodegeneration, and cognitive decline in sporadic Alzheimer's disease: a prospective cohort study. *Lancet Neurol* **12**(4) 357–367.

CASE 36 "I Have Snored All My Life and It Never Affected My Work"

Case: This 61-year-old right-handed man presented with a 3-year history of worsening memory and slowness in thinking. Working as an accountant, he first noticed his ability to process information quickly had diminished, particularly when performing calculations. Multitasking had also become more challenging. More recently, he became forgetful and more often relied on making notes, uncharacteristic for him. He reported he would eventually remember things, but usually needed a hint to do so. He did not experience any changes in language or visuospatial abilities. He denied depression, but acknowledged feeling tired most of the day, despite sleeping nine hours at night and napping for one hour on the weekends. He reported a 20-year history of polysomnogram (PSG)-confirmed obstructive sleep apnea (apnea-hypopnea index of 35, consistent with severe sleep apnea), but had not used a continuous positive airway pressure (CPAP) machine. His current medication regimen included aspirin, enalapril, and metformin. Other than obesity, his general physical examination was unremarkable. On neuropsychological evaluation, he exhibited impaired performance in repeating numbers forward and backward, as well as with Trail Making Test Part B, suggesting impaired attention and executive functions. On memory testing he showed a variable rate of learning, suggesting impaired attention and concentration. He was able to recall only 4 of the 10 words freely, but was able to recognize the rest, consistent with impairment in retrieval rather than encoding. His brain MRI showed mild subcortical white matter changes with normal hippocampal size.

Should Chronic Sleep Apnea Be Given Priority for His Cognitive Impairment?

With aging, cognitive reserve declines and the brain becomes more susceptible to many factors that affect brain function. Despite a long-standing "compensated" history, a condition that can potentially affect cognition can have a belated effect. Moreover, all potentially treatable risk factors for cognitive impairment should be considered at the initial visit.

Sleep breathing disorders (SBD) impacts cognitive function through multiple mechanisms. These include direct ones like hypoxia and sleep fragmentation, as well as indirect mechanisms, including the increase in risk for hypertension and diabetes (Rosenzweig et al., 2015). Moreover, SBD may play a direct role in the neurodegenerative process of Alzheimer disease (AD) by decreasing amyloid clearance (Wang et al., 2017). Given the treatable nature of SBD, they should be screened for in everyone with cognitive complaints.

The patient agreed to use a CPAP machine and returned to the clinic four months later reporting marked improvement in his level of alertness as well as his performance at work. He also described that he was able to concentrate better and did not require notes as much. Formal neuropsychological testing was not repeated.

Discussion

SBD range from upper respiratory resistance to sleep apnea. Their prevalence ranges from 3 percent to 17 percent in adults and increases with age (Peppard et al., 2013). However, they are more prevalent in the context of cognitive impairment: SBD is five times more common in patients with AD compared to age-matched individuals without cognitive impairment (Emamian et al., 2016).

Snoring and daytime sleepiness are the most common, symptoms of SBD. However, the subjective assessment of sleepiness is often inaccurate with chronic sleep deprivation; individuals lose the ability to perceive that they are sleepy and may misinterpret the ability to fall asleep easily or anywhere as a sign of being a "good sleeper." Proxy reports may be more sensitive, such as observations of unintended dozing, snoring, or apnea episodes. Nocturia may be a presenting symptom; an individual with disturbed sleep will be more likely to awaken at night to urinate and treatment of sleep apnea may reduce or eliminate nighttime urination. Additionally, the fragmented sleep pattern of apnea may be perceived as insomnia and treated with sleep aids. Sleep apnea may also be present without evidence of snoring or excessive daytime sleepiness. Subjective cognitive and behavioral complaints are frequently reported, including problems with concentration, impaired memory, irritability, and depressed mood. Other symptoms include dry mouth and morning headaches.

Cognitive changes associated with SBD usually involve impairments in vigilance/attention, executive functions or memory (Zhou et al., 2016). In the presence of frontal-subcortical impairment individuals should be screened for SBD, even in the context of a clear neurodegenerative condition (Mery et al., 2017). Language ability and visuospatial function are usually unaffected (Bucks et al., 2013). The impairments of vigilance/attention strongly correlate with the severity of SBD and the degree of daytime sleepiness (Zhou et al., 2016). Memory impairments involve retrieval rather than encoding, suggesting an executive-based pattern of deficit (Naegele et al., 2006). Although performance in memory and executive function tasks does not appear to a have strong correlation with sleepiness, it does with attention (Vaessen et al., 2015). Moreover, treatment of SBD with CPAP improves cognitive performance more often among those in whom daytime sleepiness is present (Barbe et al., 2001; Zhou et al., 2016). Interestingly, individuals with OSA may perform normally on more difficult tasks, such as digit span backward or tests of sustained attention, such as Trails A. Paradoxically, under task conditions where there is greater cognitive demand, individuals with OSA may be able to rally cognitive reserve, at least for a limited period of time.

In addition to benefits on sleepiness and cognition, treatment of SBD also improves mood (Haddock and Wells, 2018). In patients with advanced dementia, SBD treatment may not substantially improve cognitive performance, but may help decrease sleep fragmentation and nighttime awakenings. The benefits of treatment also extend to better glycemic control and lower cardiovascular morbidity and mortality (cardiac or stroke) (Foldvary-Schaefer and Waters, 2017). Finally, the use of CPAP may also have direct impact in the neurodegenerative process in AD, observed in normal CSF AD biomarker profile in those treated compared to persistence of the abnormal profile in those untreated (Liguori et al., 2017).

Diagnosis: Sleep apnea–induced cognitive impairment

Tip: Sleep breathing disorders are a treatable source of cognitive impairment and neuropsychiatric symptoms. The benefits of treatment may go beyond improvement in cognitive performance, mood, and level of energy, favorably impacting blood pressure and glycemic control, and maybe lowering the risk for stroke and Alzheimer disease.

References

Barbe, F. et al. 2001. Treatment with continuous positive airway pressure is not effective in patients with sleep apnea but no daytime sleepiness. a randomized, controlled trial. *Ann Intern Med* **134**(11) 1015–1023.

Bucks, R. S., Olaithe, M. and Eastwood, P. 2013. Neurocognitive function in obstructive sleep apnoea: a meta-review. *Respirology* **18**(1) 61–70.

Emamian, F. et al. 2016. The association between obstructive sleep apnea and Alzheimer's disease: a meta-analysis perspective. *Front Aging Neurosci* **8** 78.

Foldvary-Schaefer, N. R. and Waters, T. E. 2017. Sleep-disordered breathing. *Continuum* **23**(4) 1093–1116.

Haddock, N. and Wells, M. E. 2018. The association between treated and untreated obstructive sleep apnea and depression. *Neurodiagn J* **58**(1) 30–39.

Liguori, C. et al. 2017. Obstructive sleep apnea is associated with early but possibly modifiable Alzheimer's disease biomarkers changes. *Sleep* **40**(5) zsx011 1–10.

Mery, V. P. et al. 2017. Reduced cognitive function in patients with Parkinson disease and obstructive sleep apnea. *Neurology* **88**(12) 1120–1128.

Naegele, B. et al. 2006. Which memory processes are affected in patients with obstructive sleep apnea? An evaluation of 3 types of memory. *Sleep* **29**(4) 533–544.

Peppard, P. E. et al. 2013. Increased prevalence of sleep-disordered breathing in adults. *Am J Epidemiol* **177**(9) 1006–1014.

Rosenzweig, I. et al. 2015. Sleep apnoea and the brain: a complex relationship. *Lancet Respir Med* **3**(5) 404–414.

Vaessen, T. J. A., Overeem, S. and Sitskoorn, M. M. 2015. Cognitive complaints in obstructive sleep apnea. *Sleep Med Rev* **19**(Suppl C) 51–58.

Wang, J., Gu, B. J., Masters, C. L. and Wang, Y. J. 2017. A systemic view of Alzheimer disease – insights from amyloid-beta metabolism beyond the brain. *Nat Rev Neurol* **13**(11) 703.

Zhou, J., Camacho, M., Tang, X. and Kushida, C. A. 2016. A review of neurocognitive function and obstructive sleep apnea with or without daytime sleepiness. *Sleep Med* **23** (Suppl C) 99–108.

Case: This 51-year-old right-handed woman had experienced cognitive decline for 8 years. Her husband first observed that she had difficulties finding and pronouncing words correctly (e.g., saying *bindow* instead of *window*). In addition, she had become increasingly forgetful. Her ability to communicate steadily declined, and for the past 18 months she has been unable to sustain a meaningful conversation. Although she occasionally could retrieve appropriate words, her speech often consisted of nonwords. She did not follow verbal commands, but she was able to imitate and repeat short, single words intermittently. She spent hours in front of a mirror talking to herself. She remained affectionate toward her husband and was fully dependent on him for her basic activities of daily living (i.e., feeding, bathing). She did not endorse depression or anxiety but was easily irritated. Gait was preserved with no falls. A trial of donepezil 5 mg daily years ago was discontinued due to worsening irritability. Her father was diagnosed with dementia in his forties and died at age 52. She had two older sisters and two daughters with no neurological symptoms.

On neurological examination she was alert but could not follow verbal commands. Her speech was fluent but unintelligible due to neologisms. She also exhibited echolalia (Video 37.1). Her motor and sensory examination were unremarkable. Prior workup had ruled out metabolic, infectious, and autoimmune etiologies associated with rapidly progressive dementia (see Case 34). Brain MRI showed diffuse atrophy, involving the hippocampi and posterior cingulate cortex (Figure 37.1).

Given Her Early Presentation with Language Impairment and Worsening with Cholinesterase Inhibitors, Would You Consider Genetic Testing for Frontotemporal Lobar Degeneration?

Although the advanced stage of her condition precludes her classification within a cognitive syndrome some clues can be found in her history. First, her word-finding difficulties with normal fluency would be consistent with logopenic progressive aphasia, more often associated with Alzheimer disease (AD) rather than frontotemporal lobar degeneration (FTLD). Second, the lack of significant motor and behavioral abnormalities also favors AD over FTLD. Finally, the pattern of atrophy is inconsistent with FTLD. In addition, the report of worsening irritability with cholinesterase inhibitors does not favor a diagnostic impression of FTLD over a familial form of AD.

An autosomal dominant AD genetic panel revealed the N141I presenilin 2 (*PSEN2*) mutation.

Discussion

Early-onset Alzheimer disease (EOAD) is defined as AD with a clinical onset before the age of 65 (Zhu et al., 2015). Although EOAD represents about 5 percent of all AD cases, it is the most common neurodegenerative cause of early-onset dementia in western countries (Harvey et al., 2003). Besides the age of onset, EOAD is clinically and pathologically different than LOAD (Table 37.1). Unawareness of these differences can delay the diagnosis of EOAD.

EOAD is more likely to present with nonamnestic variants of AD (e.g., posterior cortical atrophy, logopenic variant of primary progressive aphasia) compared to LOAD (Palasi et al., 2015). In addition, attention, language, executive, and visuospatial functions are affected to a greater extent, whereas semantic memory tasks and memory retrieval are relatively preserved compared with LOAD (Joubert et al., 2016; Mendez, 2019; Palasi et al., 2015). This can be attributed to the different patterns of brain atrophy. In EOAD there is a more diffuse degeneration with more prominent involvement of the frontal and less involvement of the medial temporal lobe when compared to LOAD (Aziz et al., 2017; Mendez, 2017). These differences can also be observed with fluorodeoxyglucose positron emission tomography (FDG-

Video 37.1 The examination demonstrates prominent jargon speech, neologisms, and echolalia. She is unable to follow commands.

Table 37.1 Features distinguishing early from late-onset Alzheimer disease

	EOAD	LOAD
Age of onset	< 65	≥ 65
History of head trauma	More frequent	Less frequent
Cardiovascular risk factors	Often absent	Often present
Clinical presentation	Higher frequency of nonamnestic presentations	Lower frequency of nonamnestic presentations
Motor symptoms	Myoclonus and seizures early in the course	Myoclonus and seizures may be late or absent
Pattern of neurodegeneration[a]	Generalized, including frontal regions	Predominantly temporal/hippocampal

[a] Can be observed on brain MRI or FDG-PET.

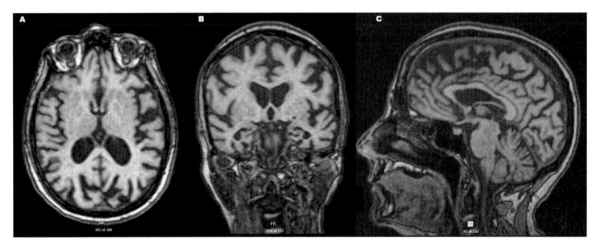

Figure 37.1 T1 brain MRI in this patient in (A) axial, (B) coronal, and (C) sagittal views. Although the atrophy is diffuse, there is greater atrophy in the hippocampi, posterior cingulate cortex, and corpus callosum.

PET) (Aziz et al., 2017; Vanhoutte et al., 2017). Amyloid scan can be a helpful tool in this population given that age does not represent a major confounder for the presence of amyloid compared to LOAD (Ossenkoppele et al., 2015). With age, there is an increase in amyloid that may or may not be associated with the major clinical syndrome. Hence, if FTD were considered in an older individual, an amyloid scan would be less useful if positive, useful only if negative. In younger individuals both a positive and negative scan would be reliable. If available, tau imaging may be considered since the distribution and burden of tau correlates with symptoms to a greater extent than amyloid (Phillips et al., 2018). Cerebrospinal fluid AD biomarkers are also helpful

in the diagnosis of AD. While differences in the concentrations of amyloid and tau among AD variants have been reported, currently there are no specific cutoff values to distinguish EAOD versus LOAD (Mendez, 2019). Finally, EOAD is associated with faster progression and higher mortality compared to LOAD (Wattmo and Wallin, 2017).

While the majority of patients with EOAD are sporadic, around 10 percent of EOAD (and 0.6 percent of all AD patients) are familial, associated with one of the three known autosomal dominant mutations: amyloid precursor protein (*APP*) (which can also be a duplication), presenilin 1 (*PSEN1*), or presenilin 2 (*PSEN2*) (Karch and Goate, 2015). Symptom onset often occurs

Table 37.2 Selected features of autosomal dominant familial Alzheimer disease

	APP	PSEN1	PSEN2
Chromosome location	21	14	1
Proportion of familial AD[a]	10%–15%	50%	5%
Onset (age, years)	40–60	35–55 (onset before 30 reported)	40–70
Disease duration before death (years [range])	8 (5–14)	8 (5–11)	11 (10–15)
Nonamnestic presentation reported	BvFTD (rare)	bvFTD Progressive aphasia Dementia with Lewy bodies Corticobasal syndrome	Progressive aphasia
Motor presentations reported	Myoclonus	Myoclonus Parkinsonism Spastic paraparesis Cerebellar ataxia	Parkinsonism
Other presentations	Epileptic seizures at onset Leukoencephalopathy Cerebral amyloid angiopathy	Epileptic seizures at onset Leukoencephalopathy Cerebral amyloid angiopathy (rare)	Cerebral amyloid angiopathy (rare)

[a] The remainder of cases remains undetermined.

between ages 30 and 60 years in the context of a family history of AD affecting at least three individuals in two or more generations. However, premature deaths from other causes may mask this pattern. In addition to cognitive presentations, autosomal dominant AD can present with other neurologic symptoms or as other syndromes, including progressive spastic paraparesis, spastic ataxia, seizures, dementia with Lewy bodies, behavioral variant frontotemporal dementia, or corticobasal syndrome (Table 37.2) (Pilotto et al., 2013). Other genetic risk factors are also associated with an increased risk of EOAD. Compared to patients with LOAD, those with EOAD have a higher frequency of two apolipoprotein E (APOE) ε4 alleles (Wattmo and Wallin, 2017). Other risk genes have been reported, and polygenic risk scores to predict EOAD are in development. However, currently their clinical utility remains limited (Chaudhury et al., 2018).

Diagnosis: Early-onset Alzheimer disease due to a *PSEN2* mutation

Tip: Alzheimer disease is the most common neurodegenerative cause of early-onset dementia. Early-onset Alzheimer disease, especially familial, is associated with a nonamnestic (or even noncognitive) presentation.

References

Aziz, A. L. et al. 2017. Difference in imaging biomarkers of neurodegeneration between early and late-onset amnestic Alzheimer's disease. *Neurobiol Aging* **54** 22–30.

Chaudhury, S. et al. 2018. Polygenic risk score in postmortem diagnosed sporadic early-onset Alzheimer's disease. *Neurobiol Aging* **62** 244.e241.

Harvey, R. J., Skelton-Robinson, M. and Rossor, M. N. 2003. The prevalence and causes of dementia in people under the age of 65 years. *J Neurol Neurosurg Psychiatry* **74**(9) 1206–1209.

Joubert, S. et al. 2016. Early-onset and late-onset Alzheimer's disease are associated with distinct patterns of memory impairment. *Cortex* **74** 217–232.

Karch, C. M. and Goate, A. M. 2015. Alzheimer's disease risk genes and mechanisms of disease pathogenesis. *Biol Psychiatry* **77**(1) 43–51.

Mendez, M. F. 2017. Early-onset Alzheimer disease. *Neurol Clin* **35**(2) 263–281.

Mendez, M. F. 2019. Early-onset Alzheimer disease and its variants. *Continuum* **25**(1) 34–51.

Ossenkoppele, R. et al. 2015. Prevalence of amyloid PET positivity in dementia syndromes: a meta-analysis. *JAMA* **313**(19) 1939–1949.

Palasi, A. et al. 2015. Differentiated clinical presentation of early and late-onset Alzheimer's disease: is 65 years of age providing a reliable threshold? *J Neurol* **262**(5) 1238–1246.

Phillips, J. S. et al. 2018. Tau PET imaging predicts cognition in atypical variants of Alzheimer's disease. *Hum Brain Mapp* **39**(2) 691–708.

Pilotto, A., Padovani, A. and Borroni, B. 2013. Clinical, biological, and imaging features of monogenic Alzheimer's disease. *Biomed Res Int* **2013** 689591.

Vanhoutte, M. et al. 2017. (18)F-FDG PET hypometabolism patterns reflect clinical heterogeneity in sporadic forms of early-onset Alzheimer's disease. *Neurobiol Aging* **59** 184–196.

Wattmo, C. and Wallin, A. K. 2017. Early- versus late-onset Alzheimer's disease in clinical practice: cognitive and global outcomes over 3 years. *Alzheimers Res Ther* **9**(1) 70.

Zhu, X.-C. et al. 2015. Rate of early onset Alzheimer's disease: a systematic review and meta-analysis. *Ann Transl Med* **3**(3) 38–38.

Case: This 67-year-old right-handed woman presented with a 2-year history of tremor and gait difficulties followed by cognitive impairment. The rest tremor appeared two years before her initial exam, followed six months later by falls and slow gait. Over the last year, she noticed difficulty maintaining her focus and frequently lost her train of thought. Word-finding impairment with frequent word substitutions emerged in addition to difficulties operating household appliances (e.g., remote control), which were not attributed to motor deficits. Her sister noticed she was forgetful and repetitive. She had experienced depression since age 17, currently managed with paroxetine 50 mg and amitriptyline 200 mg daily. In addition, she was on diazepam 10 mg daily for anxiety and zolpidem 10 mg at bedtime as a sleeping aid. On exam, she exhibited asymmetric resting tremor, bradykinesia, and rigidity. Her gait was slow with decreased stride length and impaired postural reflexes.

Montreal Cognitive Assessment (MoCA) score was 7/30 due to impairments in trail making, cube and clock drawing, naming, backward digit span, serial sevens, phonemic fluency, sentence repetition, similarities, and delayed recall (she did not recall any words freely but recognized the two in a multiple-choice format).

She was diagnosed with dementia associated with Parkinson disease (PDD).

Can We Attribute Her Cognitive Impairment to PDD?

Although the development of cognitive impairment in the context of Parkinson disease supports the diagnosis of PDD, other factors could be causing or contributing to her cognitive decline, particularly given that relatively severe cognitive decline developed within a short time. Medication side effects represent one of the most common reversible causes of cognitive impairment. A thorough review of the patient's medication list, with reevaluation to assess their risk/benefit ratio, is one of the most rewarding management strategies.

The patient was asked about her medication regimen and she reported she had been on the same regimen for at least four years.

Should This Last Piece of Information Discard the Role of Medications in Her Cognitive Decline?

Changes in pharmacokinetics and pharmacodynamics are seen in normal aging due to multiple mechanisms, including decline in hepatic and renal function, decrease in muscle mass with associated increase in body fat, and increase in age-dependent sensitivity to certain drugs (e.g., benzodiazepines, narcotics, and anticholinergic medications). These changes increase the susceptibility to medication-induced cognitive impairment. Therefore, the long-standing use of a medication that has known cognitive effects (e.g., amitriptyline, with significant anticholinergic properties) in the setting of a more recent and relatively rapid decline, should not rule out its contribution as a potential precipitant of cognitive impairment.

Discussion

Medications represent a common and often overlooked cause of cognitive impairment. Due to multiple medical problems, older individuals are often prescribed multiple medications and managed by different health care providers, putting them at increased risk for adverse effects (Kaufman et al., 2002). Use of many common over-the-counter sleep aids ("PM" medications) and allergy/antihistamines are some of the most potent anticholinergics and often overlooked in medication review. It is important to specifically ask about the use of these medications. Multiple mechanisms may account for drug-induced cognitive impairment. Anticholinergic burden (ACB) and sedation (e.g., related to antihistaminergic effects) represent the most common. Overall, the elderly are prescribed the highest number of ACB.

Beyond the well-established anticholinergic medications (e.g., oxybutynin and trihexyphenidyl) a wide variety of medicines have different degrees of anticholinergic activity (Table 38.1). Multiple scales indicating the ACB of specific drugs have been developed, with some variations among them (Villalba-Moreno et al., 2016). Anticholinergic side effects range from mild cognitive impairment to delirium. Subjects taking medications with high ACB demonstrate worse

Table 38.1 Selected medications with anticholinergic burden and recommended alternatives

Anticholinergic burden	Antidepressants	Antipsychotics	Anxiolytics/sleep aids	Bowel/Bladder medications	Others
High (ACB 3)	Tricyclic antidepressants Paroxetine	Quetiapine Olanzapine Chlorpromazine	Zolpidem Diphenhydramine[a] Hydroxyzine	Oxybutynin Tolterodine Trospium Solifenacin	Amantadine atropine Benztropine Cyclobenzaprine Meperidine Carbamazepine Oxcarbazepine
Mild–moderate (ACB 1–2)	Trazodone Fluoxetine Mirtazapine Duloxetine	Risperidone Haloperidol Ziprasidone	Benzodiazepines	Loperamide	Furosemide Atenolol Digoxin Morphine Prednisone
Recommended alternatives	Sertraline Venlafaxine	None	Trazodone	Mirabegron	

[a] Included in many over-the-counter medications, especially "PM" labeled.

performance in global cognitive function, processing speed and declarative memory (Lechevallier-Michel et al., 2005; Mulsant et al., 2003; Nebes et al., 2005; Papenberg et al., 2017). Higher ACB burden directly correlates with poorer cognitive performance in older adults (Gray et al., 2015; Mulsant et al., 2003). However, even medicines with minor anticholinergic properties may contribute to cognitive decline in some cases. The cognitive impairment associated with heart failure, "cardiac delirium," is due in part to the common cocktail of digoxin, furosemide, warfarin, and propranolol. In addition, medications with ACB have been associated with impairments in balance, mobility, and activities of daily living (Cao et al., 2008; Hilmer et al., 2009). Medications with sedative effects may impair attention and cause anterograde amnesia (Buffett-Jerrott and Stewart, 2002). Similar to those with ACB, cognitive adverse effects may range from mild to agitated delirium, which emerge more frequently in the older population. However, a scale with the sedative burden of individual medications has not been developed yet.

The impact in cognition of medications with ACB and sedative effects may manifest after years of sustained use, due to age-related changes already discussed. Prolonged use has also been associated with brain structural changes, including reduced total cortical volume, reduced temporal lobe thickness, and increased lateral and inferior lateral ventricular volume (Risacher et al., 2016). These changes directly correlated with the ACB score. Also, medications with ACB and sedative effects may directly increase the risk for dementia, mostly Alzheimer disease, a risk that decreases with medication discontinuation (Billioti de Gage et al., 2014; Carriere et al., 2009).

Given that she was on multiple medications with ACB and sedative effects, zolpidem was replaced with melatonin, paroxetine replaced with sertraline, and amitriptyline tapered and discontinued. She switched from diazepam to clonazepam 0.5 mg daily, as needed, for anxiety. In addition, she remained on her prior levodopa dosage of 100 mg QID. When she returned to the clinic after eight months, she described marked improvements in her functional abilities, level of energy, alertness, processing speed, memory, and mood. Her alternate-form repeat MoCA was 28/30, missing points only in trail making and failing to freely recalling one word.

Diagnosis: Medication-induced cognitive impairment in Parkinson disease, suggesting Parkinson disease dementia

Tip: A complete accounting of the medication list is necessary in all patients. Medications with anticholinergic or sedative burden may contribute to cognitive or behavioral impairment and could create a clinical picture indistinguishable from a neurodegenerative form of dementia.

References

Billioti de Gage, S. et al. 2014. Benzodiazepine use and risk of Alzheimer's disease: case-control study. *BMJ* 349 g5205.

Buffett-Jerrott, S. E. and Stewart, S. H. 2002. Cognitive and sedative effects of benzodiazepine use. *Curr Pharm Des* 8(1) 45–58.

Cao, Y. J. et al. 2008. Physical and cognitive performance and burden of anticholinergics, sedatives, and ACE inhibitors in older women. *Clin Pharmacol Ther* 83(3) 422–429.

Carriere, I. et al. 2009. Drugs with anticholinergic properties, cognitive decline, and dementia in an elderly general population: the 3-city study. *Arch Intern Med* 169 (14) 1317–1324.

Gray, S. L. et al. 2015. Cumulative use of strong anticholinergics and incident dementia: a prospective cohort study. *JAMA Intern Med* 175(3) 401–407.

Hilmer, S. N. et al. 2009. Drug burden index score and functional decline in older people. *Am J Med* 122(12) 1142–1149.

Kaufman, D. W. et al. 2002. Recent patterns of medication use in the ambulatory adult population of the United States: the Slone survey. *JAMA* 287(3) 337–344.

Lechevallier-Michel, N. et al. 2005. Drugs with anticholinergic properties and cognitive performance in the elderly: results from the PAQUID Study. *Br J Clin Pharmacol* 59(2) 143–151.

Mulsant, B. H. et al. 2003. Serum anticholinergic activity in a community-based sample of older adults: relationship with cognitive performance. *Arch Gen Psychiatry* 60(2) 198–203.

Nebes, R. D. et al. 2005. Serum anticholinergic activity, white matter hyperintensities, and cognitive performance. *Neurology* 65(9) 1487–1489.

Papenberg, G. et al. 2017. Anticholinergic drug use is associated with episodic memory decline in older adults without dementia. *Neurobiol Aging* 55 27–32.

Risacher, S. L. et al. 2016. Association between anticholinergic medication use and cognition, brain metabolism, and brain atrophy in cognitively normal older adults. *JAMA Neurol* 73(6) 721–732.

Villalba-Moreno, A. M. et al. 2016. Systematic review on the use of anticholinergic scales in poly pathological patients. *Arch Gerontol Geriatr* 62 1–8.

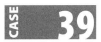

Cognitive Impairment and Blood Pressure Fluctuations

Contributed by Dr. David Riley, Cleveland, Ohio, USA

Case: This 86-year-old right-handed man with a 4-year history of Parkinson disease dementia (PDD) presented for follow-up with his wife, who reported a substantial decline. He was diagnosed with Parkinson disease (PD) five years prior and progressive cognitive impairment emerged three years later. At the visit, she described increasingly frequent episodes of unresponsiveness. These episodes would begin with the patient feeling tired, followed by a period of immobile unresponsiveness associated with glazed eyes lasting up to 10 minutes. The episodes occurred most commonly after eating breakfast. He was admitted to the hospital after one such event and his systolic blood pressure (BP) was reported to be as high as 250 mmHg, and was discharged on three new antihypertensive medications (lisinopril, hydralazine, and metoprolol). After this admission his episodes became more frequent. His wife noticed that having him lie down allowed him to recover promptly from episodes of unresponsiveness. No changes had been made to his levodopa regimen, which continued to be 200 mg three times a day.

Does the Increasing Frequency of Cognitive Fluctuations Represent Worsening Dementia?

Cognitive fluctuations increase in frequency with PDD progression and are a hallmark of the related disorder dementia with Lewy bodies (DLB). However, the pattern of these episodes occurring after eating, in addition to the immediate recovery with supine positioning, suggest orthostatic hypotension (OH) as the precipitating factor. The frequency and severity of cognitive fluctuations worsened after the addition of antihypertensive medications, further supporting this hypothesis.

At the office visit he had an episode of unresponsiveness while responding to questions. His BP was 72/48 mmHg with a pulse of 70 at that time (BP five years prior was 187/121 with a pulse of 76). He lay down on the floor with his feet elevated on the chair.

He rapidly became more alert, conversant, and able to follow commands. His BP had increased to 84/56 mmHg and his pulse was 69. After three minutes in the same position his BP rose further to 124/66 mmHg with a pulse of 61. Given the significant drop in BP without a compensatory increase in heart rate, a diagnosis of neurogenic orthostatic hypotension was made.

After the gradual discontinuation of his antihypertensive medications, the frequency of his unresponsive episodes markedly decreased. However, he continued to report fatigue and lightheadedness when standing up. Increased fluid and salt intake, the use of knee-high compression stockings, and eventually the addition of midodrine (an α1-receptor agonist prodrug), provided significant benefits in his level of alertness.

Discussion

OH is defined as a systolic blood pressure decrease of at least 20 mm Hg, or a diastolic decrease of at least 10 mm Hg, within three minutes after rising from a sitting or supine to a standing position (Freeman et al., 2011). Up to 20 percent of people older than 65 years have OH (Rutan et al., 1992). Age-associated decreases in diastolic BP, in addition to impaired baroreceptor sensitivity, are potential mechanisms in normal subjects (Huang et al., 2007). OH increases the likelihood of dementia and is an independent risk factor for mortality (Veronese et al., 2015; Wolters et al., 2016).

OH may affect up to 50 percent of patients with PD (Allcock et al., 2004). Almost two-thirds of patients with PD experience systolic BP fluctuations > 100 mmHg within a 24-hour period (Tsukamoto et al., 2013). The presence of OH in PD has been associated with both worse cognitive performance and rapid motor symptom deterioration (Fereshtehnejad et al., 2015).

Patients with OH can present with a range of symptoms when standing up, but only a third recognize them. Those with reportedly asymptomatic OH (i.e., not endorsing postural lightheadedness) have been shown to have similar impairment in activities of daily living and gait function than those with symptomatic OH (Low et al., 1995; Merola et al., 2016). Lightheadedness is the most common reported symptom, followed by weakness and cognitive difficulties (Low et al., 1995). Patients with no ostensible postural changes may describe symptoms under conditions of increased orthostatic stress, such as in the postprandial state, during high ambient temperature, or following exertion (Low and Singer, 2008). In PD, patients may also report symptoms after taking levodopa, due to its vasodilating effect.

Cognitive screening tools (e.g., Mini-Mental State Examination (MMSE)) may not be sensitive enough to identify subtle cognitive deficits present in those with OH (Allcock et al., 2006). However, more in-depth assessments among those with OH reveal poorer performance on tests of sustained attention, executive abilities, and visuospatial function (Allcock et al., 2006). These deficits improve or resolve by when the patient lies down, suggesting transient, hemodynamic-related cognitive impairments (Centi et al., 2017).

Identifying that the OH is of neurogenic versus nonneurogenic etiology allows treatment to be tailored (Table 39.1) (Goldstein and Sharabi, 2009). Increases in heart rate greater than 15 bpm within three minutes of standing suggest nonneurogenic OH, while individuals with neurogenic OH exhibit no substantial change in pulse (Gibbons et al., 2017). Nonneurogenic OH may be managed by reducing or eliminating triggers (e.g., hypotension-inducing beta-blockers and diuretics) and enacting nonpharmacologic strategies, such as increasing noncaffeinated fluids and salt intake, using thigh-high compressive leg stocking, and avoiding large meals and excessive heat exposure. In persistent neurogenic OH, hypertensive agents need to be considered (Low and Tomalia, 2015). Correction of OH has been shown to reduce cognitive fluctuations, fatigue, and lightheadedness in patients with dementia (Freidenberg et al., 2013). Patients with neurogenic OH, whose autonomic dysfunction also makes them prone to supine hypertension (SH), may be placed on antihypertensive drugs, but this can aggravate OH-related symptoms, as documented in our patient. Severe nocturnal SH may warrant a bedtime dose of a short-acting antihypertensive treatment, which minimizes nocturia and early morning OH worsening due to relative hypovolemia after nocturnal diuresis (Low

and Tomalia, 2015). The clinical and cognitive impact of SH in the context of concurrent neurogenic OH has never been assessed systematically but is suspected to yield less long-term cerebro- and cardiovascular complications compared with chronic essential hypertension, which by definition is non paroxysmal (Espay et al., 2016).

Diagnosis: OH-mediated cognitive fluctuations in a patient with Parkinson disease dementia

Tip: (Neurogenic and nonneurogenic) OH is a highly prevalent and often unrecognized cause of cognitive fluctuations in PD. Although neurodegenerative disorders themselves may be associated with dysautonomia, nonneurogenic OH triggers include antihypertensive medications, heat exposure, large carbohydrate meals, and dehydration.

References

Allcock, L. M. et al. 2006. Orthostatic hypotension in Parkinson's disease: association with cognitive decline? *Int J Geriatr Psychiatry* **21**(8) 778–783.

Allcock, L. M., Ullyart, K., Kenny, R. A. and Burn, D. J. 2004. Frequency of orthostatic hypotension in a community based cohort of patients with Parkinson's disease. *J Neurol Neurosurg Psychiatry* **75**(10) 1470–1471.

Centi, J. et al. 2017. Effects of orthostatic hypotension on cognition in Parkinson disease. *Neurology* **88**(1) 17–24.

Espay, A. J. et al. 2016. Neurogenic orthostatic hypotension and supine hypertension in Parkinson's disease and related synucleinopathies: prioritisation of treatment targets. *Lancet Neurol* **15**(9) 954–966.

Fereshtehnejad, S. M. et al. 2015. New clinical subtypes of Parkinson disease and their longitudinal progression: a prospective cohort comparison with other phenotypes. *JAMA Neurol* **72**(8) 863–873.

Freeman, R. et al. 2011. Consensus statement on the definition of orthostatic hypotension, neurally mediated syncope and the postural tachycardia syndrome. *Clin Auton Res* **21**(2) 69–72.

Freidenberg, D. L., Shaffer, L. E., Macalester, S. and Fannin, E. A. 2013. Orthostatic hypotension in patients with dementia: clinical features and response to treatment. *Cogn Behav Neurol* **26**(3) 105–120.

Gibbons, C. H. et al. 2017. The recommendations of a consensus panel for the screening, diagnosis, and treatment of neurogenic orthostatic hypotension and associated supine hypertension. *J Neurol* **264**(8) 1567–1582.

Table 39.1 Suggested steps in the management of orthostatic hypotension

Management of orthostatic hypotension

1 – Identifying and treating reversible etiologies (nonneurogenic OH)

- Hypovolemia (e.g., dehydration, chronic blood loss, adrenal insufficiency)
- Cardiac pump failure (e.g., aortic stenosis, myocardial infarction, pericarditis)

2 – Identify medications that may be contributing to OH

- Antihypertensive agents
    - o Beta-blockers (e.g., metoprolol, labetalol, carvedilol)
    - o Alpha-1 adrenergic antagonists (e.g., tamsulosin, terazosin, prazosin)
    - o Diuretics (e.g., furosemide, hydrochlorothiazide, spironolactone)
    - o Calcium channel blockers (e.g., amlodipine, verapamil, diltiazem)
    - o Renin-angiotensin system antagonists (e.g., enalapril, captopril, losartan)
    - o Other vasodilators (e.g., hydralazine, nitrates, sildenafil)
- Dopaminergic agents (e.g., levodopa and dopamine agonists)
- Anticholinergics (e.g., atropine, glycopyrrolate, hyoscyamine)
- Tricyclic antidepressants (e.g., amitriptyline, nortriptyline, imipramine)

3 – Implement nonpharmacological measures

- Increase fluid and salt intake
- Salt tablets (up to 2 g three times a day)
- Wear compression stocking or abdominal binders
- Eat small meals
- Elevate the head of the bed (minimizes effects of supine hypertension)

4 – Start pharmacological treatment (for neurogenic OH)

Drug	Mechanism of action	Dosage
Midodrine[a]	VC – α1-adrenoreceptor-agonist prodrug	2.5–10 mg TID
Droxidopa[a]	VC – Norepinephrine prodrug	100–600 mg TID
Fludrocortisone	VE – Synthetic mineralocorticoid	0.1–1 mg QD
Pyridostigmine	SAM – Acetylcholinesterase inhibitor	30 mg BID to 60 mg TID
Domperidone	SAM – Peripheral dopamine D2 receptor antagonist	10 mg BID to 30 mg TID
Desmopressin	VE – Vasopressin analogue	100–400 µg QHS
Octreotide	VC – Somatostatin analogue	25–150 µg before meals
Indomethacin	VDI – Nonsteroidal anti-inflammatory	75–150 mg QD
Dihydroergotamine	VC – Serotonin receptor agonist	3–5 mg TID
Ephedrine	VC – α1-adrenoreceptor-agonist	15 mg TID
Yohimbine	SAM – α2-adrenoreceptor-antagonist	6 mg QD
Clonidine	VE – α2-adrenoreceptor-agonist	0.4–0.8 mg QD
Atomoxetine	SAM – norepinephrine-transporter antagonist	18–36 mg QD

5 – Start nighttime pharmacological treatment for SH, if needed

Drug	Mechanism of action	Dosage
Captopril	VD/UE – Angiotensin-converting enzyme inhibitor	25–50 mg
Clonidine	VD – α2-adrenoreceptor-agonist	0.1–0.2 mg
Hydralazine	VD – Arteriole vasodilator	10–50 mg
Losartan	VD/UE – Angiotensin II receptor antagonist	50–100 mg
Nitroglycerine patch	VD – Nitric oxide prodrug	0.1–0.2 mg/hr

Note: VC: vasoconstriction; VD: vasodilation; VDI: vasodilation inhibitor; VE: volume expansion; SAM: sympathetic activity modulator; US: urinary volume expansion.

[a] The US Food and Drug Administration approved midodrine in 1996 for "symptomatic OH" and droxidopa in 2014 "symptomatic neurogenic OH caused by primary autonomic failure (Parkinson disease, multiple system atrophy and pure autonomic failure)."

Goldstein, D. S. and Sharabi, Y. 2009. Neurogenic orthostatic hypotension: a pathophysiological approach. *Circulation* **119**(1) 139–146.

Huang, C. C. et al. 2007. Effect of age on adrenergic and vagal baroreflex sensitivity in normal subjects. *Muscle Nerve* **36**(5) 637–642.

Low, P. A. et al. 1995. Prospective evaluation of clinical characteristics of orthostatic hypotension. *Mayo Clin Proc* **70**(7) 617–622.

Low, P. A. and Singer, W. 2008. Management of neurogenic orthostatic hypotension: an update. *Lancet Neurol* 7(5) 451–458.

Low, P. A. and Tomalia, V. A. 2015. Orthostatic hypotension: mechanisms, causes, management. *J Clin Neurol* **11**(3) 220–226.

Merola, A. et al. 2016. Orthostatic hypotension in Parkinson's disease: does it matter if asymptomatic? *Parkinsonism Relat Disord* **33** 65–71.

Rutan, G. H. et al. 1992. Orthostatic hypotension in older adults. The Cardiovascular Health Study. CHS Collaborative Research Group. *Hypertension* **19**(6 Pt 1) 508–519.

Tsukamoto, T., Kitano, Y. and Kuno, S. 2013. Blood pressure fluctuation and hypertension in patients with Parkinson's disease. *Brain Behav* **3**(6) 710–714.

Veronese, N. et al. 2015. Orthostatic changes in blood pressure and mortality in the elderly: the Pro.V.A Study. *Am J Hypertens* **28**(10) 1248–1256.

Wolters, F. J. et al. 2016. Orthostatic hypotension and the long-term risk of dementia: a population-based study. *PLoS Med* **13**(10) e1002143.

Case: This 68-year-old right-handed woman experienced a 6-year history of memory impairment. Her family first noticed she had difficulty recalling significant dates and recipes. She became more repetitive and forgetful, particularly for recent events and conversations. Impaired orientation and ability to follow directions prevented her from driving. In the two years prior to her evaluation, she became withdrawn and irritable, and exhibited left hemibody stiffness, leg dragging, and decreased arm swing. When asked about her ability to use tools, she noticed she no longer could use her left hand, attributing this to being right-handed.

On examination she exhibited left-predominant rigidity, bradykinesia and myoclonus. Her gait was remarkable for left leg dystonia and decreased left arm swing (Video 40.1). She showed impaired stereognosis and graphesthesia on the left hand. There were some spatial and timing errors during left-hand praxis testing. Montreal Cognitive Assessment (MoCA) score was 17/30 due to impairments in trail making, cube drawing, backward digit span, phonemic fluency, abstraction, and delayed recall (she recalled no words freely and recognized four when multiple choices were given). Her brain MRI revealed asymmetric cortical atrophy affecting predominantly the right frontal, parietal, and temporal lobes (Figure 40.1). Given the asymmetric parkinsonism, dystonia, and cortical sensory loss in the context of this imaging finding, the diagnosis of corticobasal syndrome (CBS) was made.

Should We Assume Corticobasal Degeneration (CBD) Is the Pathology of This Patient's CBS?

CBD is the most common underlying pathology of CBS. However, other neurodegenerative diseases may present with the same syndrome, including Alzheimer disease (Table 40.1). Given the parietal cortical deficits (i.e., astereognosia and agraphesthesia) and

myoclonus, the possibility of AD as the underlying pathology should be considered. Further workup, including neuropsychological evaluation and CSF AD biomarkers, need to be considered.

A neuropsychological evaluation revealed deficits in memory encoding, semantic knowledge, and visuospatial abilities. Cerebrospinal fluid AD biomarkers showed borderline elevation of both p-tau (58.05 pg/ml), with a decrease in amyloid β-42/total tau index (ATI) (1.18). However, they did not reach the cutoff for biomarker-defined Alzheimer disease (p-tau > 68 pg/ml and ATI < 0.8).

Discussion

CBS is a syndrome characterized by the lateralized presentation of a combination of deficits localized in cortical and subcortical structures. Depending on the hemisphere most affected, cortical findings include cortical sensory loss, alien limb phenomena, apraxia, myoclonus, nonfluent aphasia, apraxia of speech, pyramidal signs, and visuospatial impairment (Hassan et al., 2011). Subcortical findings include dystonia and parkinsonism.

The most common underlying pathology in CBS is 4-repeat tauopathy, accounting for half of the cases. Among the 4-R tauopathies, corticobasal degeneration (CBD) represents 35 percent of cases, while the rest of cases include progressive supranuclear palsy (Lee et al., 2011). Although CBS is not a very common presentation of AD, up to 25 percent of CBS cases have underlying AD pathology (Armstrong et al., 2013; Lee et al., 2011).

In the context of a CBS phenotype, predicting the underlying pathology represents a significant challenge. Presentations of CBS due to tauopathy (CBS-Tau) can be indistinguishable from those due to AD (CBS-AD). However, certain features are helpful to orient the clinician when considering the most likely underlying pathology. These stem from the different patterns of neurodegeneration seen in tauopathies and AD. While the first group more often affects the prefrontal and

---

Video 40.1 The examination demonstrates asymmetric bradykinesia and freezing episodes on finger tapping and left leg dystonia when walking. On apraxia evaluation, she exhibited mild spatial and timing errors with her left hand when asked to pretend to eat soup.

Table 40.1 Reported causes of corticobasal syndrome

Sporadic neurodegenerative	Genetic neurodegenerative	Other
• Corticobasal degeneration • Progressive supranuclear palsy • Pick disease • Alzheimer disease • Dementia with Lewy bodies • TDP-43 proteinopathy • Creutzfeldt–Jakob disease	• *MAPT* gene mutation • Progranulin gene mutation • *C9orf72* gene expansion • Presenilin 1 mutation • *LRRK2* gene mutation • Spinocerebellar ataxia type 8 • Cerebrotendinous xanthomatotis	• Idiopathic basal ganglia calcification • Cerebrovascular disease • Neurosyphilis • Central pontine myelinolysis • Progressive multifocal leukoencephalopathy

Source: Adapted from Chahine et al. (2014).

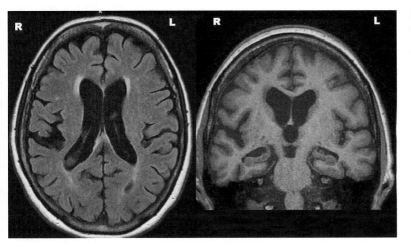

Figure 40.1 FLAIR axial and coronal brain MRI in this patient. Note the predominant right frontal, parietal, and temporal atrophy, including the hippocampi.

premotor cortex and subcortical nuclei, AD has a parietotemporal preference (Whitwell et al., 2010).

Cognitive deficits are often reported in the context of CBS (Borroni et al., 2011). Cortical deficits localizing to the parietal lobe, including visuospatial deficits, cortical sensory loss, Gerstmann syndrome and hemisensory neglect, should also raise the suspicion index for CBS-AD, in addition to logopenic aphasia (Boyd et al., 2014). On the other hand, deficits associated with frontal lobe pathology, like nonfluent aphasia, agrammatism, apraxia of speech and orobuccal apraxia, are more frequent in CBS-Tau (Hassan et al., 2011).

Motor symptoms could also assist in (imperfectly) predicting the underlying pathology. For instance, myoclonus has been documented more frequently in AD and supranuclear gaze palsy in CBS-Tau, although they are not exclusive to these groups (Hassan et al., 2011). On the other hand, parkinsonism and alien limb phenomena yielded equivocal outcomes (Borroni et al., 2011; Lee et al., 2011; Shelley et al., 2009). The

phenomenology of the alien hand syndrome can help determine the distribution of atrophy (Hassan and Josephs, 2016). For instance, the frontal or "wayward" variant is characterized by impulsive groping and manipulation of objects and the limb may not be reported as foreign; the posterior or parietal variant by levitation and a sensation of estrangement from the limb (Table 40.2).

Structural imaging supports a more frontal and focal pattern of atrophy in CBS-Tau, different to a more widespread, predominantly parietotemporal atrophy in CBS-AD (Whitwell et al., 2010). Patterns of hypometabolism on molecular imaging tend to mirror the patterns of atrophy: frontal hypometabolism suggests CBS-Tau whereas parieto-occipital and posterior cingulate hypometabolism, CBS-AD (Pardini et al., 2019).

Finally, evaluation of AD biomarkers should be considered in the evaluation of patients with CBS. These include amyloid and tau PET scan and cerebrospinal fluid biomarkers. However, it should be noted that

Table 40.2 Alien hand syndrome: classic and extended phenotypes and localization

Variant	Main features	Associated features	Common etiologies
Frontal (wayward, "pseudoalien")	"Frontal" alien hand syndrome: grasping reflex, manual groping, and utilization behavior of the *contralateral* hand	Groping, grasping, and utilization behaviors are "disobedient" or "wayward" but not truly alien	Medial frontal, supplementary motor cortex, or anterior callosum (tumors, left ACA stroke)
Callosal	Intermanual conflict and manual interference of the (usually) contralateral hand	Other disconnection syndromes: ideomotor apraxia, tactile anomia, and agraphic aphasia	Callosotomy, callosum demyelination (multiple sclerosis, Machiafava–Bignami syndrome), tumors (lipomas, gliomas, lymphoma)
Posterior ("classic" alien)	"Sensory" alien hand syndrome: withdrawal or avoidance of the *contralateral* hand	Hemianesthesia, anosognosia, hemianopia, dystonia, cortical sensory loss, and "triple ataxia" in some[a]	Parieto-occipital region lesions (AD, DLB, CBD, CJD, and PCA-distribution strokes)

[a] The posterior alien hand may be associated with "triple ataxia" in patients with extensive PCA-distribution stroke: sensory ataxia (involvement of the ventral posterolateral thalamus), cerebellar ataxia (lesion of dentatorubrothalamic tract), and optic ataxia (damage to the splenium and occipital cortex). AD: Alzheimer disease; CBD: corticobasal degeneration; CJD: Creutzfeldt–Jakob disease; DLB: dementia with Lewy bodies; PCA: posterior cerebral artery.

Source: From Rodriguez-Porcel et al. (2016).

the combination of multiple pathologies is not uncommon in CBS (Pardini et al., 2019). For example, at least 20 percent of CBD cases will also have amyloid pathology. Therefore, ascertaining the presence of one pathologic process does not rule out others. In this case, the borderline values obtained for CSF biomarkers could result from concomitant pathology or the nature of focalized pathology, restricting the "spillover" of measurable proteins into the CSF.

Diagnosis: Corticobasal syndrome associated with probable Alzheimer disease

Tip: Corticobasal syndrome can be a phenotypic manifestation of Alzheimer disease pathology. A parieto-temporal pattern of atrophy is suggestive of CBS-AD. Obtaining amyloid and tau markers is recommended.

References

Armstrong, M. J. et al. 2013. Criteria for the diagnosis of corticobasal degeneration. *Neurology* **80**(5) 496–503.

Borroni, B. et al. 2011. CSF Alzheimer's disease–like pattern in corticobasal syndrome: evidence for a distinct disorder. *J Neurol Neurosurg Psychiatry* **82**(8) 834–838.

Boyd, C. D. et al. 2014. Visuoperception test predicts pathologic diagnosis of Alzheimer disease in corticobasal syndrome. *Neurology* **83**(6) 510–519.

Chahine, L. M. et al. 2014. Corticobasal syndrome: five new things. *Neurol Clin Pract* **4**(4) 304–312.

Hassan, A. and Josephs, K. A. 2016. Alien hand syndrome. *Curr Neurol Neurosci Rep* **16**(8) 73.

Hassan, A., Whitwell, J. L. and Josephs, K. A. 2011. The corticobasal syndrome-Alzheimer's disease conundrum. *Expert Rev Neurother* **11**(11) 1569–1578.

Lee, S. E. et al. 2011. Clinicopathological correlations in corticobasal degeneration. *Ann Neurol* **70**(2) 327–340.

Pardini, M. et al. 2019. FDG-PET patterns associated with underlying pathology in corticobasal syndrome. *Neurology* **92**(10) e1121.

Rodriguez-Porcel, F. et al. 2016. Fulminant corticobasal degeneration: agrypnia excitata in corticobasal syndrome. *Neurology* **86**(12) 1164–1166.

Shelley, B. P. et al. 2009. Is the pathology of corticobasal syndrome predictable in life? *Mov Disord* **24**(11) 1593–1599.

Whitwell, J. L. et al. 2010. Imaging correlates of pathology in corticobasal syndrome. *Neurology* **75**(21) 1879–1887.

41 Another Case of Vascular Cognitive Impairment?

Contributed by Dr. Jorge Guy Ortiz Garcia and Dr. Jose Biller, Maywood, Illinois, USA

Case: This 52-year-old right-handed female presented with a 10-year history of cognitive decline, heralded by difficulty concentrating, along with mild depression and anxiety. Despite improvement of her mood with antidepressant medication, her ability to focus continued to deteriorate. Within a few years, she exhibited difficulty with multitasking, affecting her performance at work as a petrographer. She could still manage her basic activities of daily living, but they demanded more effort than before. Relevant medical history included migraines with aura and hypertension, which had been under good control for the past eight years. She was taking bupropion 450 mg and amlodipine 5 mg daily. Her family history was relevant for stroke in her mother in fifties and migraine in her mother and sister. The neurological examination was remarkable for brisk reflexes and difficulties with tandem gait. Neuropsychological evaluation revealed impairment of executive abilities, including processing speed, task switching and working memory, as well as impairments in memory encoding and retrieval. Brain MRI showed extensive, symmetric, white matter changes (Figure 41.1).

Is This Presentation Suggestive of White Matter Changes due to Vascular Disease Secondary to Hypertension?

Considering her disproportionately large burden of white matter abnormalities compared to the relatively mild hypertension, the progressive impairments in attention and executive function in the setting of confluent white matter hyperintensity also suggested a (genetic) leukoencephalopathy. Also, her cognitive function continued to deteriorate despite adequate blood pressure control with low-dose amlodipine. Critically, the involvement of the anterior temporal poles along with the external and extreme capsules, is not a recognized pattern in hypertensive encephalopathy. This pattern is consistent with cerebral autosomal dominant arteriopathy with subcortical infarcts and leukoencephalopathy (CADASIL), clinically supported here by a clinical onset in the forties and a family history of stroke and migraine.

She was found to have a mutation in the NOTCH 3 gene (520T>C), confirming the diagnosis of CADASIL.

Discussion

Cerebrovascular disease leads to cognitive impairment by two mechanisms: as a result of strategic ischemic or hemorrhagic lesions (see Case 11) or due to small-vessel disease (SVD). While the onset of symptoms and the localization of the lesion make the former easier to identify, the latter represents a twofold challenge (Skrobot et al., 2017).

First is the identification of small-vessel disease and its etiology. Although the MRI is very sensitive in the detection of white matter abnormalities, it is not very helpful in the differentiation of the underlying mechanism (Smith, 2016). In addition, the severity of white matter changes does not correlate well with the degree of cognitive impairment (Brickman et al., 2011). The presence of T2 subcortical white matter hyperintensities has a broad differential, including genetic leukoencephalopathies of pseudovascular nature and neurodegenerative conditions, such as frontotemporal lobar degeneration (Ahmed et al., 2014; Ayrignac et al., 2015). White matter hyperintensities due to vascular disease are usually accompanied by the presence of lacunar infarctions and microhemorrhages, often affecting the basal ganglia, thalamus, and internal capsule (Sarbu et al., 2016). Moreover, vascular disease can have multiple etiologies (Table 41.1) (Kanekar and

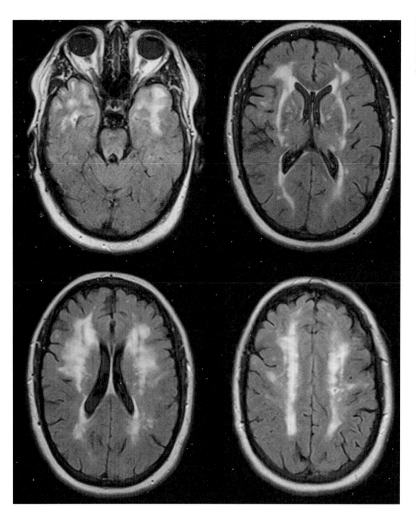

Figure 41.1 FLAIR axial brain MRI in this patient. Note the symmetric involvement of the anterior temporal poles and external and extreme capsules, characteristic of CADASIL.

Poot, 2014). While atherosclerotic SVD is the most common cause other etiologies need to be considered.

Second, the detection of vascular disease does not imply finding the cause of cognitive impairment. Determining whether the identified SVD is sufficient to account for the observed cognitive impairment is one of the most challenging tasks (Smith, 2016). In this case, clinical judgment based on the severity and location of the vascular changes was the only tool, given the lack of objective measures. Moreover, the presence or appearance of SVD or SVD-like lesions on brain MRI does not exclude concomitant neurodegenerative diseases (e.g., Alzheimer disease and frontotemporal lobar degeneration) (Gorelick et al., 2011). Finally, a stepwise progression of symptoms is typically associated with multiple discrete infarcts, although it can be present with other mechanisms as well (Espay et al., 2008).

Diagnosis: Cerebral autosomal dominant arteriopathy with subcortical infarcts and leukoencephalopathy (CADASIL)

Tip: White matter changes on brain MRI suggestive of SVD should be correlated with the severity of cognitive impairment and vascular risk factors. If discrepant, other vasculopathies, genetic leukoencephalopathies, or concomitant neurodegenerative pathologies should be considered.

References

Ahmed, R. M. et al. 2014. A practical approach to diagnosing adult onset leukodystrophies. *J Neurol Neurosurg Psychiatry* **85**(7) 770–781.

Ayrignac, X. et al. 2015. Adult-onset genetic leukoencephalopathies: a MRI pattern-based approach in a comprehensive study of 154 patients. *Brain* **138**(Pt 2) 284–292.

Table 41.1 Clinical and imaging clues distinguishing select mechanisms of cerebrovascular disease

Vasculopathy	Example	Clinical clues	Imaging clues
Atherosclerotic	Hypertension-related arteriolosclerosis	Poorly controlled vascular risk factors	WMH involving basal ganglia, thalami, internal capsule, and pons
Cerebral amyloid angiopathy	Sporadic CAA	History of hemorrhages	Multiple hemorrhages usually affecting the parietal and occipital lobe; inflammatory form is rare
Inherited vasculopathy	CADASIL	Young adults History of migraines Family history of similar symptoms	Symmetric WMH affecting the temporal pole, external capsule, and corpus callosum
Inflammatory vasculitides	Susac syndrome	Young adults Hearing loss, retinopathy, and encephalopathy	WMH involving the corpus callosum; meningeal (lepto or pachy) enhancement
Radiation therapy	Whole-brain radiation	History of radiation	Acute: contrast enhancement Late: calcification, necrosis not affecting subcortical nuclei

Note: CAA: cerebral amyloid angiopathy; CADASIL: cerebral autosomal dominant arteriopathy with subcortical infarcts and leukoencephalopathy; WMH: white matter hyperintensities.

Brickman, A. M. et al. 2011. White matter hyperintensities and cognition: testing the reserve hypothesis. *Neurobiol Aging* **32**(9) 1588–1598.

Espay, A. J. et al. 2008. Lower-body parkinsonism: reconsidering the threshold for external lumbar drainage. *Nat Clin Pract Neurol* **4**(1) 50–55.

Gorelick, P. B. et al. 2011. Vascular contributions to cognitive impairment and dementia: a statement for healthcare professionals from the American Heart Association/American Stroke Association. *Stroke* **42**(9) 2672–2713.

Kanekar, S. and Poot, J. D. 2014. Neuroimaging of vascular dementia. *Radiol Clin North Am* **52**(2) 383–401.

Sarbu, N. et al. 2016. White matter diseases with radiologic-pathologic correlation. *Radiographics* **36**(5) 1426–1447.

Skrobot, O. A. et al. 2017. The Vascular Impairment of Cognition Classification Consensus Study. *Alzheimers Dement* **13**(6) 624–633.

Smith, E. 2016. Vascular cognitive impairment. *Continuum* **22**(2) 490–509.

Case: This 77-year-old man presented with a 6-year history of worsening short-term memory and urinary urgency. He first noticed difficulties multitasking and remembering long lists, with significant benefit from cueing. He later noticed word-finding difficulties and would lose track of the topic of conversation. Around that time, he began experiencing worsening urinary urgency, followed by incontinence. Two years prior to his evaluation, his gait became increasingly slower, leading eventually to multiple falls. He also became withdrawn and more irritable. On exam, he exhibited symmetric bradykinesia, rigidity, and postural impairment. His gait was wide based with external rotation of the feet and inability to tandem walk (Video 42.1). His brain MRI was interpreted as showing asymmetric cortical atrophy with asymmetric ventriculomegaly (Image 42.1). Given an ostensible presentation with memory impairment, and suspected atrophy on imaging, Alzheimer disease (AD) was diagnosed and he was started on a treatment trial with donepezil.

Does the Clinical Presentation Fit Alzheimer Disease?

The description of multitasking-associated impaired memory and forgetfulness, with benefits from cueing, and difficulty following the thread of conversations implicated attention and executive abilities impairment rather than primary deficits in memory. These features suggested a frontal-subcortical impairment, rather than the temporal pathology typical of AD. Moreover, although gait impairment may be present in AD, it is usually subtle and not symptomatic in the early stage.

Considering the Brain MRI Pattern of Atrophy, What Alternative Diagnoses May Be Warranted to Consider?

Although the brain MRI was interpreted as showing ventriculomegaly congruent with parenchymal

atrophy (Figure 42.1), closer inspection demonstrated contralateral isolated sulcal enlargement in higher axial cuts associated with narrowing of the sulci over the cerebral convexity (Figure 42.1B), suggesting a communicating hydrocephalus disproportionate to the extent of (any true) parenchymal atrophy. Together with these imaging features, his progressive gait, urinary, and frontal-subcortical cognitive impairments supported the diagnosis of probable normal pressure hydrocephalus (NPH).

He underwent an external lumbar drainage trial for three days, in which cerebrospinal fluid (CSF) was removed round-the-clock at a rate of 10 cc/hour, resulting in improvements in gait velocity (33 percent), step length (26 percent), and urinary symptoms (Video 42.2). Both he and his family reported marked improvements in attention, processing speed, and mood, although these were not reflected in the psychometric testing to the same extent. Ventriculoperitoneal shunt (VPS) placement was therefore recommended.

Discussion

NPH is used to denote a disorder of ventriculomegaly that is associated with normal opening pressure but cannot be explained by parenchymal brain atrophy or obstructive etiologies, possibly through disruption in the balance between production and reabsorption of CSF. Ventriculomegaly may lead to disruption of periventricular white matter tracts, particularly in the frontal lobe (Lenfeldt et al., 2008). NPH is a slowly progressive disorder whose response to VPS varies due to potentially irreversible disruption to brain networks or comorbid neurodegenerative disorders that may also present with hydrocephalus on imaging (see Case 50).

The clinical presentation of NPH is associated with an insidious development of gait abnormalities first, bladder dysfunction later, and cognitive impairment

---

Video 42.1 The examination shows a mildly wide-based gait with external rotation of the feet.

Video 42.2 Shown is an examination after the placement of the drainage. Note the improvement in speed and turning when compared to the previous video.

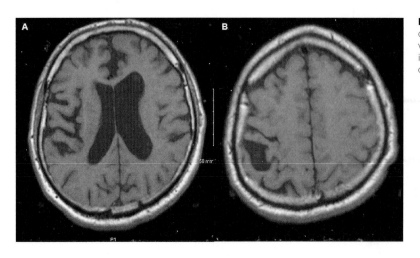

Figure 42.1 T1-weighted axial brain MRI demonstrating (A) asymmetric ventriculomegaly and (B) contralateral isolated sulcal dilation in the presence of otherwise narrow sulci.

last (Williams and Relkin, 2013). The first symptom of NPH may not be gait impairment, however, as seen in our case. Therefore, it is important to consider NPH even if it doesn't follow the "classic" progression (Mori et al., 2012). A true cognitive presentation, however, is exceptional: of 41 patients meeting criteria for NPH at the Mayo Clinic, only 1 of the 6 with sustained benefit from shunting at 3 years had cognitive impairment at presentation (Klassen and Ahlskog, 2011). The clinical presentation must be supported by the presence of communicating hydrocephalus without substantial parenchymal volume loss (ex vacuo hydrocephalus).

The Evans' ratio is the most commonly used screening measurement for hydrocephalus. It is defined as the ratio between the widest diameter of the frontal horns and the widest diameter of the inner table of the cranium on the same axial slice (Figure 42.2A) (Mori et al., 2012). NPH guidelines use an Evans' ratio threshold of ≥0.3 to define hydrocephalus (Williams and Relkin, 2013). The reliability of this index has been questioned based on the multiple variables that affect the acquisition of the measurements (e.g., level of section level; imaging protocol), and its weak correlation with ventricular volumes (Toma et al., 2011). The third ventricle is also usually enlarged, while the fourth ventricle may not be (Greitz, 2004). The sagittal views of the third and fourth ventricle should be carefully investigated for evidence of obstructive hydrocephalus.

In some patients, CSF may accumulate in the subarachnoid space causing dilatation in sulci and fissures, which may be mistaken for parenchymal atrophy, as in our case. Dilatation of the subarachnoid space may present with two patterns: disproportionately enlarged subarachnoid space hydrocephalus (DESH) and

isolated sulcal dilation (Mori et al., 2012). DESH can be recognized by the enlargement of the subarachnoid spaces in the Sylvian fissures and basal cisterns, with narrowing of the subarachnoid spaces over the high cerebral convexity and medial surface (Figure 42.2) (Hashimoto et al., 2010). The presence of DESH is a useful indicator of abnormal CSF distribution. A tight convexity with narrowed subarachnoid spaces, unlike the enlarged sulci seen in lower cuts, is a clue to distinguish this pseudoatrophic pattern of NPH from the hydrocephalus that may accompany some neurodegenerative dementias, in which there is true parenchymal atrophy (Hashimoto et al., 2010; Kitagaki et al., 1998). Isolated sulcal dilation or "sulcal entrapment" is usually observed in the medial aspect of the convexity of the brain and can be identified by marked narrowing of the adjacent sulci (Figure 42.2C) (Kitagaki et al., 1998).

Also, unlike the case in neurodegenerative disorders, non–ex vacuo hydrocephalus causes expansion of the ventricular system, which affects the morphology of adjacent structures. The corpus callosum bows out in sagittal views (Figure 42.2D), and may form an acute callosal angle on coronal views (Figure 42.2E) (Cagnin et al., 2015; Ishii et al., 2008; Lane et al., 2001).

Assessment of hydrocephalus must always include inspection of parenchymal integrity on brain MRI. Hippocampal atrophy and widening of the hippocampal sulci are mild compared to AD (Savolainen et al., 2000). Thin T2-weighted hyperintense bands extended around the ventricular system, including the ventricular horns, suggest transependymal flow (42.2f). These changes are usually difficult to differentiate from white matter lesions of presumed vascular etiology, with which they are assumed to coexist (Malm et al., 2013). The

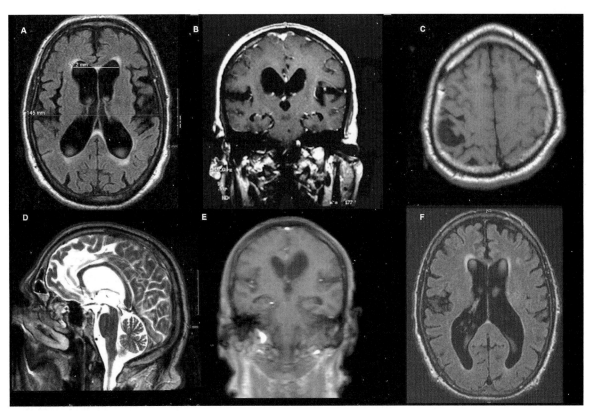

Figure 42.2 MRI changes suggestive of normal pressure hydrocephalus: (A) Evans' higher than 0.3; (B) DESH suggested by the presence of ventriculomegaly associated with dilation of Sylvian fissure but narrow sulci in the convexity of the brain; (C) isolated sulcal dilation with tight adjacent sulci; (D) bowing of the corpus callosum; (E) formation of an acute callosal angle on coronal sequences; and (F) T2-hyperintense bands surrounding the ventricular system, suggestive of transependymal flow.

hydrocephalic presentation of neurodegenerative disorders must be taken into account when considering a shunt (see Case 50) (Starr et al., 2014). Indeed, alternative or additional neurological diagnosis were given to 5 of 12 shunted "NPH" patients in the Mayo Clinic series (none of whom had sustained improvement with VPS) (Klassen and Ahlskog, 2011).

Diagnosis: Normal pressure hydrocephalus

Tip: Careful assessment of the ventricular system and surrounding parenchyma is warranted to distinguish NPH from hydrocephalic presentations of neurodegenerative disorders. The presence of sulcal dilatation in the context of tight brain convexity suggests "entrapped" CSF rather than true parenchymal atrophy.

References

Cagnin, A. et al. 2015. A simplified callosal angle measure best differentiates idiopathic-normal pressure hydrocephalus from neurodegenerative dementia. *J Alzheimers Dis* **46**(4) 1033–1038.

Greitz, D. 2004. Radiological assessment of hydrocephalus: new theories and implications for therapy. *Neurosurg Rev* **27**(3) 145–165; discussion 166–147.

Hashimoto, M., Ishikawa, M., Mori, E. and Kuwana, N. 2010. Diagnosis of idiopathic normal pressure hydrocephalus is supported by MRI-based scheme: a prospective cohort study. *Cerebrospinal Fluid Res* **7** 18.

Ishii, K. et al. 2008. Clinical impact of the callosal angle in the diagnosis of idiopathic normal pressure hydrocephalus. *Eur Radiol* **18**(11) 2678–2683.

Kitagaki, H. et al. 1998. CSF spaces in idiopathic normal pressure hydrocephalus: morphology and volumetry. *AJNR Am J Neuroradiol* **19**(7) 1277–1284.

Klassen, B. T. and Ahlskog, J. E. 2011. Normal pressure hydrocephalus: how often does the diagnosis hold water? *Neurology* **77**(12) 1119–1125.

Lane, J. I., Luetmer, P. H. and Atkinson, J. L. 2001. Corpus callosal signal changes in patients with obstructive hydrocephalus after ventriculoperitoneal shunting. *AJNR Am J Neuroradiol* **22**(1) 158–162.

Lenfeldt, N. et al. 2008. Idiopathic normal pressure hydrocephalus: increased supplementary motor activity accounts for improvement after CSF drainage. *Brain* **131** (Pt 11) 2904–2912.

Malm, J. et al. 2013. Influence of comorbidities in idiopathic normal pressure hydrocephalus – research and clinical care. A report of the ISHCSF task force on comorbidities in INPH. *Fluids Barriers CNS* **10**(1) 22.

Mori, E. et al. 2012. Guidelines for management of idiopathic normal pressure hydrocephalus: second edition. *Neurol Med Chir* **52**(11) 775–809.

Savolainen, S. et al. 2000. MR imaging of the hippocampus in normal pressure hydrocephalus: correlations with cortical Alzheimer's disease confirmed by pathologic analysis. *AJNR Am J Neuroradiol* **21**(2) 409–414.

Starr, B. W., Hagen, M. C. and Espay, A. J. 2014. Hydrocephalic Parkinsonism: lessons from normal pressure hydrocephalus mimics. *J Clin Mov Disord* **1** 2.

Toma, A. K., Holl, E., Kitchen, N. D. and Watkins, L. D. 2011. Evans' index revisited: the need for an alternative in normal pressure hydrocephalus. *Neurosurgery* **68**(4) 939–944.

Williams, M. A. and Relkin, N. R. 2013. Diagnosis and management of idiopathic normal-pressure hydrocephalus. *Neurol Clin Pract* **3**(5) 375–385.

43 Parkinsonism, Ataxia, and Cognitive Impairment after Radiation Therapy

Case: This 60-year-old woman presented with a 6-year history of bilateral hand tremor and progressive gait impairment. She first noticed bilateral hand tremor when holding objects, followed by balance impairment, slow walking with foot dragging, and a tendency to fall forward. Within four years, she required a wheelchair for ambulation. She endorsed initial short-term memory affecting her ability to process information, which accelerated in the last year. Two years prior to the onset of her symptoms she had received chemotherapy (carboplatin and etoposide) with prophylactic whole-brain radiation as treatment for lung cancer.

There was no family history of cognitive impairment or movement disorders. Two of her sister's children had intellectual disability. She did not have children due to infertility. On exam she exhibited symmetric bradykinesia with mild action tremor, but no rigidity. She was unable to walk unaided, exhibiting a wide-based gait with difficulties in turning and freezing of gait (Video 43.1). Her Montreal Cognitive Assessment (MoCA) score was 12/30, with errors in orientation, visuospatial/executive tasks, attention, phonemic fluency, and delayed recall (she was unable to recall any words unaided, but recognized 3/5 words when multiple choices were given). Her brain MRI demonstrated diffuse atrophy with moderate leukoencephalopathy (Figure 43.1). Given the recent history of brain radiation, her symptoms and MRI findings were considered supportive of postradiation cognitive impairment.

Can Her Symptoms Be Truly Attributed to Postradiation Effects?

The contribution of whole-brain radiation to her symptoms is uncertain. The presence of ataxia and tremor at onset followed by cognitive impairment is atypical for what has been described in post brain-radiation injury (Greene-Schloesser et al., 2012). Post brain-radiation injury can have a delayed presentation with progressive dementia, dysarthria, and seizures fewer than six months after treatment, with the prevalence of cognitive impairment increasing with age (Greene-Schloesser et al., 2012). In our patient, however, parkinsonism was the predominant early motor feature, which is atypical for post-brain radiation injury. In addition, she had family history of interest (nephews with intellectual disability), and the leukoencephalopathic changes involved the callosal splenium, also atypical. Therefore, whole-brain radiation is not tenable as the unifying etiology.

What Alternative Diagnosis Should We Consider?

Progressive ataxia, action tremor, and parkinsonism associated with cognitive impairment in the context of family history of intellectual disability and personal history of infertility strongly suggest fragile X–associated tremor-ataxia syndrome (FXTAS), a possibility admittedly far more common in males. The FLAIR and T2-weighted hyperintensity in the splenium of the corpus callosum (Figure 43.1) is supportive. She was evaluated for CGG expansions in the *FMR1* gene and was found to be a carrier of 82 and 132 CGG expansions in the *FMR1* gene, under the premutation range, which confirms the diagnosis of FXTAS.

Discussion

FXTAS is a neurodegenerative syndrome associated with premutation range CGG expansions (55 to 200) in the fragile X mental retardation 1 gene (*FMR1*) (Hagerman and Hagerman, 2016). FXTAS affects primarily men > 55 years of age and represents the most severe neurologic syndrome associated with *FMR1* premutations. The prevalence of premutation carriers is around 1:150 among women and 1:450 among men. However, the penetrance is lower in women with approximately 40–75 percent of men carriers developing FXTAS compared to only 16–20 percent in women

---

Video 43.1 The examination demonstrates symmetric bradykinesia with mild action tremor and subtle limb ataxia. Gait is wide based with increased difficulties in turning.

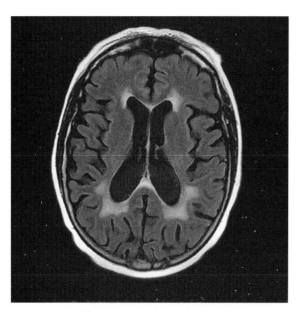

Figure 43.1 FLAIR axial brain MRI in this patient. Note the confluent white matter hyperintensities in the periventricular and corpus callosum splenium.

Table 43.1 Common comorbidities in FXTAS

Common comorbidities in FXTAS
Attention-deficit hyperactivity disorder
Obsessive-compulsive disorder
Sleep apnea
Hypertension
Hypothyroidism
Autonomic neuropathy
Migraine
Premature ovarian failure

Note: These disorders are increased among *FMR1* premutation carriers. Those that may contribute to cognitive impairment are noted in bold.

carriers (Hagerman and Hagerman, 2016). The proposed mechanisms include the random inactivation of one X chromosome in every somatic cell through the process of lyonization, and a protective effect of the unaffected X chromosome (Hagerman and Hagerman, 2016; Hall et al., 2014; Seltzer et al., 2012). In the case presented, the presence of two premutated alleles is the likely explanation for her more severe presentation. The classic description of the syndrome includes progressive action tremor, cerebellar ataxia, and cognitive impairment (Hagerman et al., 2001). Tremor, usually presenting as symmetric high-amplitude action tremor and often misattributed as essential tremor, is typically followed by truncal ataxia and falls (Leehey et al., 2007). The greater the CGG repeat size the more severe the cognitive impairment, tremor, and ataxia, with a magnitude of milder severity in women (Leehey et al., 2008). Mild parkinsonian features, manifesting as generalized bradykinesia, rigidity, and slow gait, with modest response to levodopa, may be present, particularly in women (Leehey, 2009). Peripheral neuropathy is a feature observed in almost all patients (Leehey, 2009).

Executive function, particularly inhibition and working memory, is the cognitive domain initially and predominantly affected (Grigsby et al., 2014). When memory becomes affected, encoding and

recognition are normal, suggesting a retrieval deficit due to frontal network dysfunction (Yang et al., 2014). While mild anomia may be present in early stages, language is otherwise normal, as are visuospatial abilities (Grigsby et al., 2014). Cognitive impairment tends to evolve into dementia to a greater extent in older males (Seritan et al., 2008; Seritan et al., 2013). Behavioral features include moria (i.e., euphoria) and increased anxiety, while depression is less common (Hagerman and Hagerman, 2016). The cognitive and behavioral changes observed in FXTAS correspond to those described in the cerebellar cognitive affective syndrome. Comorbid neurodegenerative pathology, including Alzheimer and Lewy body disease has been reported in FXTAS, although the prevalence of dual pathology is unknown (Tassone et al., 2012). Premutation carriers, with or without FXTAS, are at an increased risk for multiple medical conditions, some of which may contribute to cognitive impairment, and therefore should be considered during the evaluation (Table 43.1) (Hagerman and Hagerman, 2016).

Brain imaging is invariably abnormal in FXTAS, showing generalized brain atrophy, with or without atrophy of the corpus callosum and cerebellum (Figure 43.2A) (Apartis et al., 2012). White matter changes are a common finding, presenting as T2-weighted hyperintensities involving the periventricular region and the pons (Hagerman and Hagerman, 2016). Bilateral middle cerebellar peduncle (MCP) hyperintensities (Figure 43.2B) are seen in 60 percent of patients, although it can also be seen in other disorders, such as the cerebellar type of multiple system atrophy (MSA-C) (Brunberg et al., 2002). Corpus

Table 43.2 Selected etiologies leading to MCP sign and increased signal in the corpus callosum splenium

Bilateral MCP sign	Corpus callosum splenium sign
Neurodegenerative	**Neurodegenerative**
• FXTAS	• FXTAS
• Multiple system atrophy, cerebellar type	
Demyelinating	**Demyelinating**
• Multiple sclerosis	• Multiple sclerosis
• *Progressive multifocal leukoencephalopathy*	• *Progressive multifocal leukoencephalopathy*
• *Acute disseminated encephalomyelitis*	• *Acute disseminated encephalomyelitis*
Dysmyelinating	**Dysmyelinating**
• X-linked adrenoleukodystrophy	• X-linked adrenoleukodystrophy
	• Metachromatic leukodystrophy
Vascular	**Vascular**
• *Posterior reversible encephalopathy syndrome*	• *Posterior reversible encephalopathy syndrome*
• Bilateral anterior inferior cerebellar artery infarcts	• Bilateral posterior cerebral artery infarct
Toxic-metabolic	**Toxic-metabolic**
• *Osmotic demyelination syndrome*	• Marchiafava–Bignami disease
• *Hepatic encephalopathy*	• *Amphetamine abuse*
• Wilson disease	• *Cyclosporine toxicity*
• *Heroin abuse*	• *Phenytoin toxicity*
• *Toluene abuse*	• *Metronidazole toxicity*
• *Methotrexate toxicity*	
Neoplastic	**Neoplastic**
• Primary CNS lymphoma	• Primary CNS lymphoma
• Astrocytoma	• Glioblastoma multiforme
Infectious	**Others**
• Viral infections	• *Hypoxic-ischemic encephalopathy*
• Whipple disease	• *Postepileptic*
• Lyme disease	• *Viral infections*
	• *Postventricular shunting*

Note: Potentially transient lesions are shown in italics.

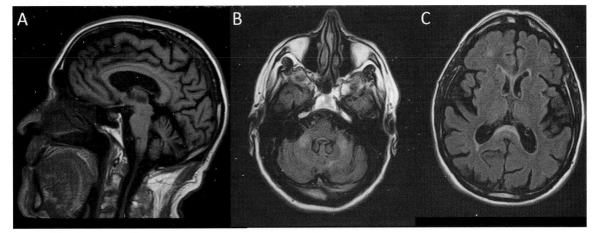

Figure 43.2 MRI changes seen in FXTAS: (A) cortical atrophy associated with cerebellar and callosal atrophy; (B) bilateral middle cerebellar peduncle hyperintensity; (C) hyperintensity of the corpus callosum splenium.

callosum splenium hyperintensities (Figure 43.2C) may be more frequently observed in women, but appear to be less specific for the diagnosis (Table 43.2) (Apartis et al., 2012).

The fragile X mental retardation 1 gene (*FMR1*) on chromosome X normally has 5 to 40 CGG repeats in the 5′ untranslated region (Hagerman, 2013). Expansions beyond the normal range lead to two distinct pathological processes depending on the number of repeats. The presence of a full mutation (i.e., > 200 CGG repeats) is associated with epigenetic silencing of the gene (Hagerman and Hagerman, 2016). These subjects with fragile X syndrome (FXS) are predominantly male and exhibit nonprogressive intellectual disability or autism spectrum disorder during childhood (Hagerman and Hagerman, 2016). Expansions ranging between 55 and 200 repeats, the premutation range, result in an increase in mRNA production, which is associated with gain-of-function toxicity (Hagerman and Hagerman, 2016). CGG expansions are considered unstable, leading to an increase in the repeats in the children of premutation carriers compared to their affected parents. Therefore, FXTAS should be considered in elderly men with ataxia and action tremor with grandchildren affected by intellectual disability or autism spectrum disorder (FXTAS begets FXS). In women, a similar presentation, in addition to a history of early ovarian failure, should raise the suspicion for FXTAS.

Diagnosis: Fragile X–associated tremor/ataxia syndrome

Tip: Although more common in men, FXTAS should be considered in women with ataxia, action tremor, parkinsonism, and cognitive impairment, and a family history of intellectual disability, autism spectrum disorder, or early ovarian failure. MRI may show hyperintensities in the MCP and splenium of the corpus callosum.

References

Apartis, E. et al. 2012. FXTAS: new insights and the need for revised diagnostic criteria. *Neurology* **79**(18) 1898–1907.

Brunberg, J. A. et al. 2002. Fragile X premutation carriers: characteristic MR imaging findings of adult male patients with progressive cerebellar and cognitive dysfunction. *AJNR Am J Neuroradiol* **23**(10) 1757–1766.

Greene-Schloesser, D. et al. 2012. Radiation-induced brain injury: a review. *Front Oncol* **2** 73.

Grigsby, J. et al. 2014. The cognitive neuropsychological phenotype of carriers of the FMR1 premutation. *J Neurodev Disord* **6**(1) 28.

Hagerman, P. 2013. Fragile X–associated tremor/ataxia syndrome (FXTAS): pathology and mechanisms. *Acta Neuropathol* **126**(1) 1–19.

Hagerman, R. J. and Hagerman, P. 2016. Fragile X–associated tremor/ataxia syndrome – features, mechanisms and management. *Nat Rev Neurol* **12**(7) 403–412.

Hagerman, R. J. et al. 2001. Intention tremor, parkinsonism, and generalized brain atrophy in male carriers of fragile X. *Neurology* **57**(1) 127–130.

Hall, D. A. et al. 2014. Emerging topics in FXTAS. *J Neurodev Disord* **6**(1) 31.

Leehey, M. A. 2009. Fragile X–associated tremor/ataxia syndrome: clinical phenotype, diagnosis, an treatment. *J Investig Med* **57**(8) 830–836.

Leehey, M. A. et al. 2008. FMR1 CGG repeat length predicts motor dysfunction in premutation carriers. *Neurology* **70**(16 Pt 2) 1397–1402.

Leehey, M. A. et al. 2007. Progression of tremor and ataxia in male carriers of the FMR1 premutation. *Mov Disord* **22**(2) 203–206.

Seltzer, M. M. et al. 2012. Prevalence of CGG expansions of the FMR1 gene in a US population-based sample. *Am J Med Genet B Neuropsychiatr Genet* **159b**(5) 589–597.

Seritan, A., Cogswell, J. and Grigsby, J. 2013. Cognitive dysfunction in FMR1 premutation carriers. *Curr Psychiatry Rev* **9**(1) 78–84.

Seritan, A. L. et al. 2008. Dementia in fragile X–associated tremor/ataxia syndrome (FXTAS): comparison with Alzheimer's disease. *Am J Med Genet B Neuropsychiatr Genet* **147b**(7) 1138–1144.

Tassone, F. et al. 2012. Neuropathological, clinical and molecular pathology in female fragile X premutation carriers with and without FXTAS. *Genes Brain Behav* **11**(5) 577–585.

Yang, J. C. et al. 2014. ERP abnormalities elicited by word repetition in fragile X–associated tremor/ataxia syndrome (FXTAS) and amnestic MCI. *Neuropsychologia* **63** 34–42.

Case: This 85-year-old right-handed man presented with a 5-year history of memory difficulties. His daughter described a slowly progressive decline in his ability to recall recent events. Initially, he repeated stories and frequently misplaced items. Within the prior two years, he forgot appointments and started adding notes to calendars. Otherwise, he remained very independent and active, exercising daily. He exhibited no motor or personality changes. The patient was not concerned about his difficulties and attributed them to normal aging. His only medication was tamsulosin for prostatic hyperplasia. His neurological exam was normal except for a Montreal Cognitive Assessment (MoCA) score of 25/30 due to impairments in delayed recall (he recalled one word freely; could not name the others even after category or multiple-choice cues) and orientation to time. Brain MRI showed bilateral hippocampal atrophy, disproportionate to atrophy elsewhere (Figure 44.1). He was suspected to have mild cognitive impairment due to Alzheimer disease (AD). As part of his involvement in a research study, he underwent an amyloid scan, which was normal. A subsequent lumbar puncture to evaluate CSF AD biomarkers showed borderline elevation of total tau but normal beta-amyloid and phosphorylated tau.

Given the Lack of AD Biomarkers, Are You Attributing This to Normal Aging?

The normal values in CSF beta-amyloid and p-tau ruled out Alzheimer disease (McKhann et al., 2011). However, elevation in total tau, even if borderline, suggests a neurodegenerative process. While dementia with Lewy bodies can also exhibit hippocampal atrophy, this is usually seen later in the course (Chow et al., 2012). Suspected non-Alzheimer disease pathophysiology (SNAP) is the term applied to individuals with normal levels of brain beta-amyloid but in whom biomarkers of neurodegeneration (e.g., structural MRI) are abnormal (Jack et al., 2016). This can be secondary to other pathologies different than AD, including TDP-43 proteinopathies and tauopathies (Table 44.1). Whether these pathologic findings are the result of normal aging or a pathologic process remains debatable. However,

given the degree of atrophy and the progression of symptoms, a pathologic neurodegenerative process appears to be more likely in this case.

Discussion

AD biomarkers can be classified into two categories: neurodegeneration and disease-specific markers (i.e., beta-amyloid and p-tau) (Jack et al., 2016; Jack et al., 2018). The former group includes elevated total tau (t-tau) in CSF, hypometabolism in temporal–parietal regions assessed by FDG-PET, and medial temporal lobe (MTL) atrophy assessed by MRI. However, of all biomarkers these imaging studies are the least specific for AD (Fotuhi et al., 2012). First, AD can present with other patterns of neurodegeneration (e.g., posterior cortical atrophy). Second, temporoparietal hypometabolism and MTL atrophy can be observed in the absence of AD and be associated with other neurodegenerative and nonneurodegenerative processes.

The term hippocampal sclerosis describes neuronal loss and gliosis affecting the hippocampus and the associated structures. The hippocampus is very susceptible to anoxic/hypoxic injury. Cerebrovascular disease and anoxia have been identified as independent factors in hippocampal atrophy even if they do not lead to stroke or anoxic events (Fotuhi et al., 2012). Examples include obstructive sleep apnea, hypertension, diabetes, autoimmune disorders, and cardiac arrest (Fotuhi et al., 2012; Lu et al., 2017). Temporal lobe epilepsy manifesting in childhood or early adulthood has also been associated with hippocampal sclerosis, which is usually asymmetric or unilateral (Tai et al., 2018).

In the context of neurodegeneration, TDP-43 proteinopathies, such as hippocampal sclerosis associated with frontotemporal lobar degeneration (FTLD), limbic associated TDP-43 encephalopathy (LATE), and tauopathies, such as argyrophilic grain disease and primary age-related tauopathies (previously known as tangle dominant dementia), can present with hippocampal atrophy early in the course of the disease (Table 44.1). Early involvement of hippocampus can lead to a primarily amnestic pattern of cognitive impairment clinically indistinguishable from AD during early stages. However, in AD there is a significantly greater decline

Table 44.1 Select neurodegenerative causes of hippocampal atrophy.

Disorder	Pathology	Associated findings	Comments
Hippocampal sclerosis associated to FTLD	TDP-43 type A	FTD syndrome plus anterograde amnesia Motoneuron findings Family history	Consider genetic testing for *progranulin* and *C9orf72*
Limbic associated TDP-43 encephalopathy	TDP-43	Isolated amnesia	Common in elderly patients
Argyrophilic grain disease	4 R tauopathy	Slow progression Changes in emotion or personality	Can lead to hippocampal atrophy in the context of PSP or CBD
Primary age-related tauopathy	3 R/4 R tauopathy	Slow progression Pathology restricted to temporal lobes	Previously known as tangle dominant dementia
Pick disease	3 R tauopathy	FTD syndrome	bvFTD is the most common presentation
Chronic traumatic encephalopathy	Perivascular tauopathy and TDP-43 proteinopathy	History of head trauma	Associated with depression, suicidality

Note: CBD: corticobasal degeneration; FTD: frontotemporal dementia (syndrome); bvFTD: behavioral variant of FTD; FTLD: frontotemporal lobar degeneration (pathology), PSP: progressive supranuclear palsy.

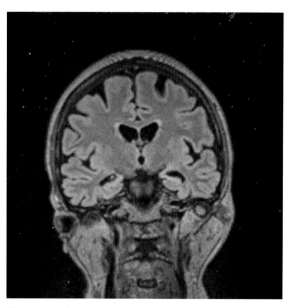

Figure 44.1 FLAIR coronal brain MRI in this patient. Note bilateral hippocampal atrophy.

in cognition, including memory, language, and visuospatial abilities, when compared to other neurodegenerative causes of hippocampal atrophy (Smirnov et al., 2019). Unfortunately, neither clinical criteria nor biomarkers currently exist for these processes (Jicha and Nelson, 2019). Exam findings or family history suggestive of frontotemporal dementia (e.g., behavioral variant

or progressive aphasia) or motor neuron disease, should raise the concern of hippocampal atrophy as a manifestation of a pathogenic neurodegenerative process. Genetic testing, including *progranulin* mutations and *C9orf72* expansions, should be considered. Tau imaging may be considered, if available, which if positive would be suggestive of underlying primary age-related tauopathy. Finally, although these are currently considered separate entities, they may coexist with other neurodegenerative processes, like AD, affecting their presentation and course (Josephs et al., 2008; Josephs et al., 2014). Moreover, they have been also reported in autopsies of subjects without overt dementia, creating a debate on their pathogenicity (Jicha and Nelson, 2019).

There was no family history of cognitive, behavioral or other neurologic diseases. He refused further testing.

Diagnosis: Suspected non-Alzheimer disease pathophysiology (SNAP)

Tip: Progressive, primarily amnestic, cognitive impairment with hippocampal atrophy but normal AD biomarkers suggest underlying tauopathies and TDP-43 proteinopathies.

References

Chow, N. et al. 2012. Comparing hippocampal atrophy in Alzheimer's dementia and dementia with Lewy bodies. *Dement Geriatr Cogn Disord* **34**(1) 44–50.

Fotuhi, M., Do, D. and Jack, C. 2012. Modifiable factors that alter the size of the hippocampus with ageing. *Nat Rev Neurol* **8** 189.

Jack, C. R., Jr. et al. 2016. A/T/N: an unbiased descriptive classification scheme for Alzheimer disease biomarkers. *Neurology* **87**(5) 539–547.

Jack, C. R., Jr. et al. 2016. Suspected non-Alzheimer disease pathophysiology: concept and controversy. *Nat Rev Neurol* **12**(2) 117–124.

Jack, C. R., Jr. et al. 2018. NIA-AA research framework: toward a biological definition of Alzheimer's disease. *Alzheimers Dement* **14**(4) 535–562.

Jicha, G. A. and Nelson, P. T. 2019. Hippocampal sclerosis, argyrophilic grain disease, and primary age-related tauopathy. *Continuum* **25**(1) 208–233.

Josephs, K. A. et al. 2008. Abnormal TDP-43 immunoreactivity in AD modifies clinicopathologic and radiologic phenotype. *Neurology* **70**(19 Pt 2) 1850–1857.

Josephs, K. A. et al. 2014. TDP-43 is a key player in the clinical features associated with Alzheimer's disease. *Acta Neuropathol* **127**(6) 811–824.

Lu, J. Q., Steve, T. A., Wheatley, M. and Gross, D. W. 2017. Immune cell infiltrates in hippocampal sclerosis: correlation with neuronal loss. *J Neuropathol Exp Neurol* **76**(3) 206–215.

McKhann, G. M. et al. 2011. The diagnosis of dementia due to Alzheimer's disease: recommendations from the National Institute on Aging-Alzheimer's Association workgroups on diagnostic guidelines for Alzheimer's disease. *Alzheimers Dement* **7**(3) 263–269.

Smirnov, D. S. et al. 2019. Trajectories of cognitive decline differ in hippocampal sclerosis and Alzheimer's disease. *Neurobiol Aging* **75** 169–177.

Tai, X. Y. et al. 2018. Review: neurodegenerative processes in temporal lobe epilepsy with hippocampal sclerosis: clinical, pathological and neuroimaging evidence. *Neuropathol Appl Neurobiol* **44**(1) 70–90.

Case: This 70-year-old right-handed woman presented with a 2-year history of slowly worsening cognition, then with more recent abrupt decline. She noted increasing difficulty recalling recent events and coming up with words. Over the last month, her family reported that she became slow in her thinking and easily confused. About a week prior to this assessment, she had been found on the floor unresponsive and taken to the emergency room, where she had a witnessed seizure. Metabolic abnormalities and infections were ruled out. A lumbar puncture showed elevated protein (80 mg/dl) but no other abnormalities. Her brain MRI without contrast showed asymmetric subcortical and periventricular T2 hyperintensities (Figure 45.1). She was started on levetiracetam 500 mg BID. Since then, she continued to decline but did not have further seizures. On examination, she exhibited bradyphrenia and fluctuating alertness. Montreal Cognitive Assessment (MoCA) score was 15/30 due to errors in trail making, clock drawing, backward numbers, serial sevens, phonemic fluency, delayed recall (she recalled two words freely, and recognized one when multiple choices were given) and orientation to date and day of the week.

What Might the Best Next Step Be?

An inflammatory process needs to be considered given the subacute progression of cognitive impairment, the development of seizures, the increase in CSF protein, and the asymmetric confluent subcortical white matter changes on brain MRI. The diagnostic workup would benefit from obtaining a brain MRI scan with contrast, as well as a paraneoplastic panel (see Case 17).

Repeat brain MRI on the next day included a susceptibility weighted imaging (SWI) sequence (a variant of the gradient-echo sequence, not included in the previous MRI) showing multiple susceptibility foci, suggestive of hemosiderin deposition (Figure 45.2).

How Does This Imaging Abnormality Help?

The presence of multiple hemosiderin deposits suggests microhemorrhages, most likely from cerebral amyloid angiopathy (CAA). Given the clinical and CSF changes, the most likely diagnosis is CAA-

related inflammation, which may be amenable to treatment with immunosuppression.

She was started on methylprednisolone 1000 mg daily for five days, followed by 60 mg of prednisone daily tapered over two weeks. Her level of alertness and cognition improved, although without return to baseline. Three months later, her MoCAs score had improved to 24/30, missing points for serial sevens, phonemic fluency and delayed recall (she recalled two words freely and the other three with category clues).

Discussion

Cerebral amyloid angiopathy is a vasculopathy characterized by deposits of amyloid within small to medium blood vessels of the brain and leptomeninges (Table 45.1). Sporadic cases of CAA are often seen in the elderly, including approximately 12 percent of patients over the age of 85 (Greenberg and Vonsattel, 1997). Carriers of the ApoE2 or E4 alleles are at a greater risk for CAA-related hemorrhage than those with only the most common ApoE3 allele (Charidimou et al., 2017). In addition, autosomal dominant mutations in the *APP* (amyloid precursor protein) gene can lead to earlier onset of CAA, with symptoms presenting in the early fifties (Wermer and Greenberg, 2018).

The most common clinical manifestation of CAA is spontaneous lobar hemorrhage, more often affecting the posterior brain regions either symmetrically or asymmetrically. The risk of hemorrhage is high in CAA and recurrent hemorrhages usually arise close to the initial hemorrhage (Rosand et al., 2005). Small cortical subarachnoid hemorrhages may occur, followed by hemosiderin deposition, known as cortical superficial siderosis (Wermer and Greenberg, 2018). The corresponding neurologic deficits depend on the localization and size of the hemorrhage. In addition, transient neurologic symptoms are often reported by patients and described as brief, stereotyped spells of either positive (e.g., paresthesia, jerking) or negative (e.g., weakness, aphasia) symptoms which can spread over contiguous body parts (Charidimou et al., 2012). These are thought to be due to vasospasm caused by cortical subarachnoid hemorrhage and superficial siderosis. However, these episodes can be sometimes mistaken as seizures or ischemic events.

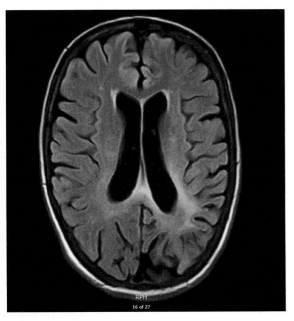

Figure 45.1 Axial fluid-attenuated inversion recovery (FLAIR) brain MRI in this patient. Note asymmetric, confluent white matter hyperintensities.

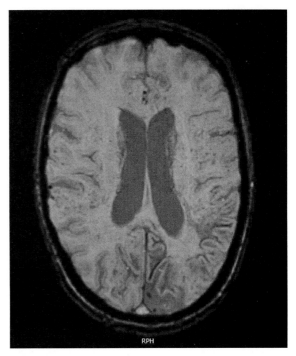

Figure 45.2 Axial susceptibility weighted imaging (SWI) brain MRI in this patient. The multiple areas of susceptibility, suggestive of hemorrhages.

Besides recurrent hemorrhages, CAA can present with an acute inflammatory process presenting with acute or subacute cognitive decline, known as CAA-related inflammation (Kinnecom et al., 2007). Other features include headache, focal neurological signs and seizures (Eng et al., 2004). Brain MRI shows patchy or confluent hyperintensities on FLAIR or T2 weighted MRI sequences in addition to lobar microhemorrhages (Auriel et al., 2016). These may be associated with leptomeningeal or parenchymal contrast enhancement, but their presence is not part of the diagnostic criteria (Auriel et al., 2016). Acute immunosuppressive treatment to prevent progression and aim at reversion of at least some of the deficits is recommended in these cases. Treatment response is variable but only a small proportion returns to their baseline (Eng et al., 2004).

Cognitive impairment is a common feature of CAA. Impairment in processing speed and executive functions seem to be primarily affected, whereas episodic memory may be relatively spared (Charidimou et al., 2017). Concomitant Alzheimer disease (AD) pathology is common but not invariably present (Arvanitakis et al., 2011). In both AD and CAA, brain amyloid on PET imaging is increased and CSF β42 amyloid is decreased. However, CSF β40, t-tau, and p-tau are all lower in CAA compared to AD, suggesting that AD is more likely when t-tau and especially p-tau are higher. These CSF profile findings are congruous with the pathologic hallmarks of CAA, which include predominant vascular deposition of Aβ40 rather than Aβ42, and variable presence of tau-containing lesions, especially in patients with symptomatic CAA presenting with hemorrhage. Higher lobar microbleed counts, white matter hyperintensities volume, and cortical superficial siderosis (CAA MRI markers) correlate with decreasing Aβ40 concentration. Overall neuronal degeneration indicated by t-tau and cortical tangle formation indicated by p-tau are higher in AD.

Definitive diagnosis of CAA can only be done by postmortem brain evaluation. Microhemorrhages on gradient-echo weighted (GRE) or susceptibility weighted imaging (SWI) imaging strongly suggests CAA (Greenberg, 1998).

Management of CAA hinges on preventing further hemorrhages. In patients with hypertension, tighter blood pressure control is warranted. Anticoagulants and antiplatelets are discouraged as they increase the risk of hemorrhage. However, anticoagulants and antiplatelets may be needed in specific situations, like atrial fibrillation, although this is an area of controversy (Charidimou et al., 2018).

Table 45.1 Diagnostic criteria for cerebral amyloid angiopathy and cerebral amyloid angiopathy-related inflammation

Probable CAA	**Clinical data and MRI or CT demonstrating**
	Multiple hemorrhages restricted to lobar, cortical, or cortical-subcortical regions (cerebellar hemorrhage allowed), **OR** single lobar, cortical, or cortical-subcortical hemorrhage and focal or disseminated superficial siderosis[a]
	Age ≥ 55 years
	Absence of other cause of hemorrhage or superficial siderosis
Possible CAA	**Clinical data and MRI or CT demonstrating**
	Single lobar, cortical, or cortical-subcortical hemorrhage, **OR** focal or disseminated superficial siderosis[a]
	Age ≥ 55 years
	Absence of other cause of hemorrhage or superficial siderosis
Probable CAA-related inflammation	Age ≥ 40 years
	Presence of more than one of the following clinical features: headache, decrease in consciousness, behavioral change, or focal neurological signs and seizures; the presentation is not directly attributable to an acute ICH
	MRI shows unifocal or multifocal WMH lesions (corticosubcortical or deep) that are asymmetric and extend to the immediately subcortical white matter; the asymmetry is not due to past ICH
	Presence of more than one of the following corticosubcortical hemorrhagic lesions: cerebral macrobleed, cerebral microbleed, or cortical superficial siderosis
	Absence of neoplastic, infectious, or other cause
Possible CAA-related inflammation	Age ≥ 40 years
	Presence of more than one of the following clinical features: headache, decrease in consciousness, behavioral change, or focal neurological signs and seizures; the presentation is not directly attributable to an acute ICH
	MRI shows WMH lesions that extend to the immediately subcortical white matter
	Presence of more than one of the following cortico-subcortical hemorrhagic lesions: cerebral macrobleed, cerebral microbleed, or cortical superficial siderosis
	Absence of neoplastic, infectious, or other cause

Note: Definite and probable CAA with supporting pathology criteria require full postmortem examination and pathologic tissue, respectively. ICH: intracerebral hemorrhage; WMH: white matter hyperintensity.

*Superficial siderosis is defined as focal when it is restricted to three or fewer sulci; when it affects four or more sulci, it is considered disseminated.

Source: Adapted from Linn et al. (2010) and Auriel et al. (2016).

Diagnosis: Cerebral amyloid angiopathy-related inflammation

Tip: When evaluating abrupt or stepwise cognitive decline associated with subcortical white matter changes, consider the potentially treatable cerebral amyloid angiopathy-related inflammation. Microhemorrhages are best observed on GRE and SWI sequences.

References

Arvanitakis, Z. et al. 2011. Cerebral amyloid angiopathy pathology and cognitive domains in older persons. *Ann Neurol* **69**(2) 320–327.

Auriel, E. et al. 2016. Validation of clinicoradiological criteria for the diagnosis of cerebral amyloid angiopathy-related inflammation. *JAMA Neurol* **73**(2) 197–202.

Charidimou, A. et al. 2012. Spectrum of transient focal neurological episodes in cerebral amyloid angiopathy: multicentre magnetic resonance imaging cohort study and meta-analysis. *Stroke* **43**(9) 2324–2330.

Charidimou, A. et al. 2017. Emerging concepts in sporadic cerebral amyloid angiopathy. *Brain* **140**(7) 1829–1850.

Charidimou, A. et al. 2018. Cerebral amyloid angiopathy, cerebral microbleeds and implications for anticoagulation decisions: the need for a balanced approach. *Int J Stroke* **13** (2) 117–120.

Eng, J. A. et al. 2004. Clinical manifestations of cerebral amyloid angiopathy-related inflammation. *Ann Neurol* **55** (2) 250–256.

Greenberg, S. M. 1998. Cerebral amyloid angiopathy: prospects for clinical diagnosis and treatment. *Neurology* **51** (3) 690–694.

Greenberg, S. M. and Vonsattel, J. P. 1997. Diagnosis of cerebral amyloid angiopathy: sensitivity and specificity of cortical biopsy. *Stroke* **28**(7) 1418–1422.

Kinnecom, C. et al. 2007. Course of cerebral amyloid angiopathy-related inflammation. *Neurology* **68**(17) 1411–1416.

Linn, J. et al. 2010. Prevalence of superficial siderosis in patients with cerebral amyloid angiopathy. *Neurology* **74** (17) 1346–1350.

Rosand, J. et al. 2005. Spatial clustering of hemorrhages in probable cerebral amyloid angiopathy. *Ann Neurol* **58**(3) 459–462.

Wermer, M. J. H. and Greenberg, S. M. 2018. The growing clinical spectrum of cerebral amyloid angiopathy. *Curr Opin Neurol* **31**(1) 28–35.

46 I Don't Know When to Stop

Case: This 59-year-old right-handed man exhibited unusual behavioral changes. He had been diagnosed with Parkinson disease (PD) four years ago. Since then, he was benefiting motorically from pramipexole, gradually increased to 1 mg three times a day. While he felt there were no problems, his wife reported that over the past year he became more withdrawn. She reported that he no longer played tennis on Saturdays, a lifelong tradition, nor did he ride his motorcycle, which he always loved doing. Previously a very social person, he did not participate in social activities and preferred to stay at home. He was spending most of his time playing games on the computer, most of them for money, something he had never done before. His wife noticed he was now sleeping less as he played until late hours. They could not tell how much money had been spent in these games. He continued to work, but his supervisor noticed a decline in his performance which he attributed to spending a significant amount of time playing on the computer. His wife thought it was due to depression, even if his motor abilities were fine overall. Although he denied feeling sad, he tried sertraline titrated to 100 mg qd with no benefit. On exam, he exhibited mild resting tremor, rigidity and bradykinesia, more evident on the left. Besides decreased left arm swing, his gait was normal. Montreal Cognitive Assessment (MoCA) score was 27/30 due to errors in trail making, cube copying and phonemic word fluency.

Do You Attribute This to the Apathy or Depression?

In this case, gambling on the computer was interpreted as a way of filling up the time left from abandoning other hobbies and interests. However, since he fixated on only one activity and couldn't disengage in order to sleep, an impulse control disorder is a more plausible explanation. The dopamine agonist, pramipexole, is the most likely cause and should be tapered down.

The nature of impulse control disorders (ICDs) and the possible association with dopamine agonists

was explained to the patient and his wife. After listing other manifestations of ICDs, his wife identified another likely example; he purchased items that he didn't really need, including a motorcycle helmet and speakers for the house.

Pramipexole was tapered down slowly and discontinued. During the tapering process his tremor worsened, which resolved with the addition of carbidopa/levodopa. After being off pramipexole for 10 days he was no longer gambling or engaging in excessive online shopping.

Discussion

Behavioral changes in PD can be disease-related or complications of treatment. Impulsive-compulsive behaviors (ICBs) is a group of disorders characterized by disruptive, repetitive, behaviors without forethought or consideration of the potential consequences (Evans et al., 2019; Weintraub and Claassen, 2017). ICBs include ICDs and dopamine dysregulation syndrome (DDS), both associated with dopaminergic replacement therapy (Table 46.1) (Bereau et al., 2018). These behavioral changes are underreported by patients and families, in part due to embarrassment or limited awareness. They are also often overlooked by the clinician. Given their disruptive consequences and treatable nature, it is imperative to routinely monitor for the presence of ICBs in any PD patients on dopaminergic medications.

ICDs are characterized by the failure to resist an impulse (also described as drive, urge or temptation) to perform a pleasurable activity with eventually negative consequences to the person or others (Weintraub et al., 2015). These activities are performed in a repetitive and excessive manner, to the extent they interfere in major areas of life functioning (Weintraub et al., 2015). Four major ICDs have been reported in PD: gambling, hypersexuality, compulsive shopping and binge eating. Compulsive sexual behavior is more common in males, whereas compulsive buying and binge eating more prevalent in women, reflecting imbalances also seen in the general population. ICDs

Table 46.1 Selected features of impulsive-compulsive behaviors associated with dopaminergic medication

	Features	Categories and examples
Impulse control disorders	Excessive engagement in pleasurable activities Thinking excessively or having urges to engage in the activity that is difficult to control Engagement in activity is disruptive (e.g., affecting work performance or finances)	**Gambling**: casinos, internet gambling, lotteries, scratch tickets, sports, slot or poker machines, or betting among friends) **Sexual behavior**: making sexual demands on others, promiscuity, prostitution, change in sexual orientation, masturbation, internet or telephone sexual activities, or pornography) **Buying**: buying excessively **Eating**: eating larger amounts or different types of food than in the past, more rapidly than normal, until feeling uncomfortably full, or when not hungry
Other impulsive-compulsive behaviors	Excessive engagement in seemingly purposeless activities May not be disruptive	Hobbyism Punding Hoarding
Dopamine dysregulation syndrome	Excessive intake of dopaminergic medication leading to motor and behavioral side effects Self-increase in dosage Report of reduced efficacy justifying the dose increases	Severe dyskinesia and dystonia Neuropsychiatric fluctuations (hypomania during on and dysphoria during the perceived off-states; objectively, patients are in a nearly uninterrupted on-state)

are more common in patients taking dopamine agonists. Whether the risk of developing an ICD is related to the dose of a dopamine agonist remains under debate due to conflicting reports (Bastiaens et al., 2013; Weintraub et al., 2010). ICD may also occur with rasagiline, levodopa or amantadine (Weintraub et al., 2010). Risk factors to develop ICDs include younger age, male sex, early-onset PD, and history of gambling, alcoholism, impulsive traits, or cigarette smoking (Weintraub and Claassen, 2017).

DDS can be understood as an "addiction" to short-acting dopaminergic medications, levodopa and apomorphine (Giovannoni et al., 2000). This is characterized by compulsive self-medication with inappropriately high doses of dopaminergic medication in the face of reported loss of drug benefit. Increased levodopa induces severe peak-dose dyskinesia and neuropsychiatric fluctuations, typically with hypomania during the on-drug state and dysphoria, depression, irritability or anxiety during the perceived off-drug states, similar to some drug withdrawal syndromes (Bereau et al., 2018).

In addition, to ICDs and DDS, other related phenomena identified in PD are recognized. Punding is a repetitive, purposeless activity, focused on specific items or activities (e.g., collecting, arranging, or taking apart objects or constantly reorganizing the objects in cabinet). Punding is driven by pleasure, not followed by a sense of relief after the behaviors, which is different from obsessive-compulsive disorder (Spencer et al., 2011). Hobbyism is similar to punding but activities are usually more complex, like reading or working on complex projects. Hoarding can emerge, leading to unsafe or unsanitary living conditions (Weintraub et al., 2015).

The approach to ICBs and related disorders starts with education of the patient and their caregivers about the potential risks of dopaminergic therapies at the time these therapies are being considered, providing directions on how to identify ICBs and emphasizing the potentially treatable nature. Once therapy is stated, the emergence of these symptoms needs to be monitored periodically and forever (Antonini et al., 2016). There are several screening tools for ICBs, including the Questionnaire for Impulsive-Compulsive Disorders in Parkinson Disease (QUIP), that also has a rating scale version available (QUIP-RS) (Weintraub et al., 2009; Weintraub et al., 2012). If a disruptive ICB has been identified, changes in dopaminergic therapy are warranted. Tapering or decreasing the dose of dopamine agonists in ICDs and short-acting levodopa agents in DDS to level where the disruptive behaviors are not present is the first step in the management. A slow taper, particularly of dopamine agonists, is recommended in order to avoid dopamine agonist withdrawal syndrome (DAWS). Symptoms of withdrawal include anxiety, including panic attacks, depression, fatigue, pain and drug cravings (Rabinak and Nirenberg, 2010). A compensatory increase in levodopa dosage using other medications may be required to address these or any worsening of motor symptoms. In the case of ICDs, other strategies include amantadine (although it has also been associated with ICDs, albeit less commonly than dopamine agonists), naltrexone and cognitive behavioral therapy (Weintraub and Claassen, 2017). Deep brain stimulation, when leading to significant decreases in dopaminergic medication is associated with improvements in ICD symptoms (Weintraub and Claassen, 2017).

Diagnosis: Impulse control disorder due to pramipexole

Tip: In patients with Parkinson disease on dopaminergic medications, particularly a dopamine agonist, education about the risk of impulse control disorders is critical. Periodic, ongoing screening is warranted.

References

Antonini, A. et al. 2016. Impulse control disorder related behaviours during long-term rotigotine treatment: a post hoc analysis. *Eur J Neurol* **23**(10) 1556–1565.

Bastiaens, J., Dorfman, B. J., Christos, P. J. and Nirenberg, M. J. 2013. Prospective cohort study of impulse control disorders in Parkinson's disease. *Mov Disord* **28**(3) 327–333.

Bereau, M. et al. 2018. Hyperdopaminergic behavioral spectrum in Parkinson's disease: a review. *Rev Neurol* **174** (9) 653–663.

Evans, A. H. et al. 2019. Scales to assess impulsive and compulsive behaviors in Parkinson's disease: critique and recommendations. *Mov Disord* **34**(6) 791–798.

Giovannoni, G. et al. 2000. Hedonistic homeostatic dysregulation in patients with Parkinson's disease on dopamine replacement therapies. *J Neurol Neurosurg Psychiatry* **68**(4) 423–428.

Rabinak, C. A. and Nirenberg, M. J. 2010. Dopamine agonist withdrawal syndrome in Parkinson disease. *Arch Neurol* **67**(1) 58–63.

Spencer, A. H., Rickards, H., Fasano, A. and Cavanna, A. E. 2011. The prevalence and clinical characteristics of punding in Parkinson's disease. *Mov Disord* **26**(4) 578–586.

Weintraub, D. and Claassen, D. O. 2017. Impulse control and related disorders in Parkinson's disease. *Int Rev Neurobiol* **133** 679–717.

Weintraub, D. et al. 2015. Clinical spectrum of impulse control disorders in Parkinson's disease. *Mov Disord* **30**(2) 121–127.

Weintraub, D. et al. 2009. Validation of the questionnaire for impulsive-compulsive disorders in Parkinson's disease. *Mov Disord* **24**(10) 1461–1467.

Weintraub, D. et al. 2010. Impulse control disorders in Parkinson disease: a cross-sectional study of 3090 patients. *Arch Neurol* **67**(5) 589–595.

Weintraub, D. et al. 2012. Questionnaire for Impulsive-Compulsive Disorders in Parkinson's Disease Rating Scale. *Mov Disord* **27**(2) 242–247.

Weintraub, D. et al. 2010. Amantadine use associated with impulse control disorders in Parkinson disease in cross-sectional study. *Ann Neurol* **68**(6) 963–968.

Case: This 76-year-old man returned to the clinic, brought by his daughter for monitoring of his progressive memory impairment. Five years previously, neuropsychological evaluation revealed memory encoding deficits and brain MRI showed asymmetric hippocampal atrophy. With a diagnosis of probable Alzheimer disease, he was started on rivastigmine, gradually increased to a dose of 6 mg BID. The family noticed better thinking and less forgetfulness for six months, but he continued to decline thereafter. He went on to have difficulty dressing and bathing and experienced delusions of theft. After five years of treatment with rivastigmine, his daughter wondered if it should be discontinued.

Should We Consider Discontinuation of Cholinesterase Inhibitors at Certain Progression Threshold?

Cholinesterase inhibitors and memantine are considered symptomatic rather than disease-modifying therapy. This means that even if the symptoms improve the neurodegenerative process continues, which ultimately translate to symptomatic worsening. However, this does not mean the agents do not continue to provide benefit. In this case, caution over discontinuing rivastigmine is warranted as the patient is exhibiting mild delusions, which could worsen with discontinuation.

The patient did not have any side effects, delusions were mild, and the patient preferred to continue the medication. Therefore, no changes were made.

Discussion

Despite how frequently this question comes up in the clinic, there is no consensus on how to address it. Discontinuation of cholinesterase inhibitors (ChEI) is easier to enact in the presence of adverse effects (e.g., nausea, diarrhea, anorexia, tremor, vivid dreaming and urinary incontinence). However, how to proceed when the benefits are not perceived remains a matter of debate given the lack of consistent results and of long-term studies (Howard et al., 2012; Scarpini et al., 2011). In practice, we suggest discouraging the discontinuation of ChEI for lack of perceived benefit unless issues related to cost or adverse effects are involved. However,

an individualized approach needs to be used. This should start by explaining to patients and their families that these medications are symptomatic and not disease-modifying therapies. Therefore, the drug may be providing symptomatic benefit even if there continues to be a decline. In addition, if not present at the time of discussion, communication issues may emerge at later stages and ChEI appear to help with word finding, discourse, and initiative to speak (Ferris and Farlow, 2013). ChEI may be discontinued in the more advanced disease stages, when hospice is being considered. At any stage, patients and their families should be informed about the potential worsening of symptoms or emergence of new ones, like aggression, after discontinuation, particularly in patients who exhibit delusions or hallucinations (Daiello et al., 2009). Abrupt worsening is discouraged given their increased risk of withdrawal (Lanctôt et al., 2015). If symptoms worsen after tapering ChEI, treatment could be restarted although it is not clear if the full benefit can be recaptured. Whether gaps on treatment affect functional outcome remains a matter of debate (Doody et al., 2001; Pariente et al., 2012). Once the decision is made to discontinue treatment, unless the medication is already at its lowest dose, it should be tapered over a period of a month with close monitoring of cognitive and behavioral symptoms.

Diagnosis: Dementia of Alzheimer type

Tip: Discontinuation of cholinesterase inhibitors due to lack of continued sustained perceived benefit is usually discouraged unless cost makes it prohibitive, or an advanced care-dependent stage is reached.

Reference

Daiello, L. A. et al. 2009. Effect of discontinuing cholinesterase inhibitor therapy on behavioral and mood symptoms in nursing home patients with dementia. *Am J Geriatr Pharmacother* 7(2) 74–83.

Doody, R. S. et al. 2001. Open-label, multicenter, phase 3 extension study of the safety and efficacy of donepezil in patients with Alzheimer disease. *Arch Neurol* **58**(3) 427–433.

Ferris, S. H. and Farlow, M. 2013. Language impairment in Alzheimer's disease and benefits of acetylcholinesterase inhibitors. *Clin Interv Aging* 8 1007–1014.

Howard, R. et al. 2012. Donepezil and memantine for moderate-to-severe Alzheimer's disease. *N Engl J Med* **366** (10) 893–903.

Lanctôt, K. et al. 2015. Predictors of worsening following cholinesterase inhibitor discontinuation trial in institutionalized persons with moderate to severe Alzheimer's disease: results of a double-blind, placebo controlled trial. *Alzheimer's Dementia* **11**(7) P520.

Pariente, A. et al. 2012. Effect of treatment gaps in elderly patients with dementia treated with cholinesterase inhibitors. *Neurology* **78**(13) 957–963.

Scarpini, E. et al. 2011. Cessation versus continuation of galantamine treatment after 12 months of therapy in patients with Alzheimer's disease: a randomized, double blind, placebo controlled withdrawal trial. *J Alzheimers Dis* **26**(2) 211–220.

Case: This 76-year-old right-handed man with an amnestic presentation, suspicious for Alzheimer disease and diagnosed 5 years earlier, returned to the clinic for follow-up. Although he initially experienced improvement with donepezil, his cognition progressively declined over the following three years. In the last six months, his wife, who was his primary caregiver, noted that he was more forgetful and repetitive. However, now when he misplaced objects (e.g., wallet, books), he became convinced that the lost objects were stolen, even when the missing items were found and shown to him. Her repeated attempts to reassure him that the objects were merely misplaced triggered agitation and confusion. No threatened or real physical aggression ensued. In the office, he had no recollection of the events. He was oriented to place and person. His speech was fluent and his discourse was circumlocutory. The remainder of the exam was unremarkable.

Should a Medication Be Considered to Address the Agitation?

Agitation is a behavior that may be experienced by a person with dementia, often in response to ineffective communication strategies or a lack of an appropriately structured environment. Unlike aggression, which involves risk of or actual physical harm to self or others, not all agitation needs medical intervention. Before considering remedies with pharmacotherapy, environmental triggers and modifiable factors should be identified and managed. In this case, the patient has a delusion of theft which likely stems from the progression of his cognitive impairment, particularly his memory loss. When he returns to the place where he habitually places an item and it is not where he expects it to be, he assumes that it must be stolen. The conclusion is not illogical, but due to gaps in memory it is being made with incomplete information. The additional lack of insight into the memory impairment affects his ability to benefit from any attempts by his wife to reorient him or provide additional information. While it is important to show the patient that the object has been found, his wife's well-intentioned explanations may actually help trigger the agitation.

What Strategies to Use?

The caregiving role is often assumed by default; most caregivers lack the type of formal education and understanding about dementia and behavior management that is demanded of professional caregivers. The first step is to investigate what the caregiver understands about the behavior and how much distress it causes. This may be best surveyed through formal assessment instruments, such as the Neuropsychiatric Inventory (NPI), which includes ratings for the effects of the behavior on both the patient and the caregiver. For simple delusions of theft or infidelity that typically occur in mid-stage Alzheimer disease, an explanation about how the memory impairment leads to the behavior can reduce the caregiver's distress at being falsely accused and provide context for other more appropriate responses (Table 48.1). The second step is to provide effective communication strategies and responses. How the caregiver reacts to a situation almost always shapes the patient's reactions. An easy mnemonic to teach is the three Rs (Table 48.1):

1. **R**ight: the patient is always right. Although incomplete, the perceptions of an Alzheimer patient are his/her reality, and caregivers need to accept this. Memory impairment often prevents demented individuals from reorientation and correction.

2. **R**eassure: verbal responses should be reassuring, addressing the core concerns without passing judgment about the truth of the situation. In case of lost items, assist in a search for them and then provide reassurance that the problem will be addressed to prevent future issues. The explanations should be short and simple.

3. **R**edirect: redirect attention to another task or topic to prevent perseverative thoughts and behaviors. Demented individuals often lack the ability to reset a thought pattern without caregiver's direction. Instruct caregivers to have a list of favorite foods, topics, or activities to use as a distracting maneuver in difficult situations.

Finally, the caregiver's well-being should be addressed during the visit. This includes referrals to caregiver education programs (often provided by

Table 48.1 Selected measures to consider in the context of behavioral symptoms in dementia

Assess the caregiver	**Use NPI or other formal behavioral survey tools to identify behaviors and their impact on caregivers** Educate caregivers about the disease and the nature of its deficits Inquire about caregivers safety, **emotional and cognitive well-being** and address, if necessary Provide resources for patient care and caregiver support groups
Steps to address agitation	Ensure safety Reconsider the situation from the perspective of the patient and make them feel they are **right**; avoid confrontation or attempting to convince the patient **Reassure** the concerns are taken into account and solutions are considered **Redirect** the focus of attention by engaging the patient of a different activity
General measures	**Establish a routine for eating, sleeping, and activity to compensate for disturbed circadian rhythms** Prioritize a familial environment (e.g., activities taking place in a room that is already familiar) Hearing and vision aids Avoid excessive sensory input
Treatment of triggers	Assess for pain Avoid dehydration Treat underlying medical conditions (e.g., infection, heart failure) Identify environmental triggers

local Alzheimer Associations), support groups, online resources, and books.

When asked about these episodes his wife endorsed being overwhelmed with his care. She also felt offended that he would accuse her of stealing and was frustrated that her constant attempts to show him he was wrong did not work. She recognized that she was impatient, which may have affected the way she responded to his accusations.

Discussion

Neuropsychiatric symptoms (NPS) are almost universally observed in dementia syndromes, regardless of the underlying etiology. These symptoms tend to be more problematic than purely cognitive symptoms, affecting the patient's but also the caregiver's health and safety (Van Den Wijngaart et al., 2007). Untreated NPS are associated with faster progression and earlier nursing home placement (Yaffe et al., 2002). While there are few well-established treatment options the common practice when NPS emerge is to resort to an antipsychotic medication. However, their efficacy is only modest in improving NPS while exposing patients to serious side effects and increased mortality and morbidity (Sink et al., 2005).

NPS may emerge as the consequence of multiple factors. These not only include the neurodegenerative process itself, but also other potentially modifiable factors (Tible et al., 2017). Focusing solely on a pharmacological approach may result in a lost opportunity (Kales et al., 2014). In addition, the adverse effects associated with use of atypical antipsychotics offset their advantages in the treatment of agitation in Alzheimer disease (Schneider et al., 2006). One approach to elucidate triggers and provide a context for addressing them involves analyzing a behavior like a detective investigating a crime (Brasure et al., 2016). An exact chronology of events, how the patient and other individuals were involved, and the environment in which the event took place should all be assessed (Kales et al., 2014).

The acute emergence of NPS and other changes in behavior raises concern for a medical change unrelated to the progression of the disease. Similar to the workup of acute dementia worsening underlying infection or iatrogenic changes should be excluded, and untreated pain and sleep impairment evaluated and managed. The decline of cognitive abilities is associated with impaired verbal communication, causing the patient to express emotions through behaviors instead of words. In addition, declining abilities may lead to a loss of purpose and boredom.

In most cases, particularly early in the disease, caregivers are family members who have not received any formal preparation to deal with the complex and burdensome task of taking care of a dementia patient. Often, caregivers use parenting models to frame their responses which inadvertently leads to infantilization and ineffective strategies to instruct or teach compensatory routines. It is also imperative to inform caregivers that behaviors and abilities may fluctuate from day to day, and that the inconsistency in performance is not an attempt by the patient to deliberately sabotage them. Some caregivers carry the burden not only of caregiving but also of being a spouse. They suffer from the emotional stress of losing a partner, a way of life, and of unrealized dreams, while being burdened with a new set of responsibilities, which, for many, they had no previous experience. Often caregivers perceive that they need to personally provide all care and do not delegate or seek assistance. Personal health and well-being are often sacrificed. Caregivers themselves may be cognitively impaired and unable to properly provide care. All of this may affect the interaction with the patient and responses to NPS. Therefore, it is important to assess the caregiver's cognitive and emotional well-being as it directly may impact patient care. Educating the caregiver to understand and manage NPS in dementia provides benefit not only to the patient, including nursing home placement, but also to the caregiver's well-being (Gitlin et al., 2008; Gitlin et al., 2010; Livingston et al., 2014).

Finally, the environment where the patient lives should be explored. Given that patients with dementia usually have difficulty processing multiple stimuli quickly, minimizing and simplifying them can prove helpful. This ranges from decluttering and eliminating sources of noise at home, breaking down tasks into simple steps and promoting socialization in smaller groups. Since demented individuals adapt poorly to change, it is best to develop and adhere to a routine for sleep, eating, and activities. Circadian rhythms malfunction in dementia and external structures need to be implemented to replace internal clocks.

In this case, the visit was devoted to counseling on the nature of the delusions and agitation, provision of concrete strategies on how to respond to agitated behaviors to avoid confrontation, and the recasting of the role of caregiver as facilitator and not educator. A referral to social work was made for longitudinal caregiver support and education.

Diagnosis: Delusion and agitation in Alzheimer disease dementia

Tip: Caregiver education is underappreciated and can have a significant impact on the patient's behavior. In the context of behavioral changes, identifying triggers and assessing the caregivers knowledge about the disease and their cognitive and emotional well-being can have a major impact. Nonpharmacological measures should be prioritized.

References

Brasure, M. et al. 2016. AHRQ comparative effectiveness reviews. In *Nonpharmacologic Interventions for Agitation and Aggression in Dementia*. Rockville, MD: Agency for Healthcare Research and Quality, pp. 1–263.

Gitlin, L. N. et al. 2008. Tailored activities to manage neuropsychiatric behaviors in persons with dementia and reduce caregiver burden: a randomized pilot study. *Am J Geriatr Psychiatry* **16**(3) 229–239.

Gitlin, L. N. et al. 2010. A biobehavioral home-based intervention and the well-being of patients with dementia and their caregivers: the COPE randomized trial. *JAMA* **304**(9) 983–991.

Kales, H. C. et al. 2014. Management of neuropsychiatric symptoms of dementia in clinical settings: recommendations from a multidisciplinary expert panel. *J Am Geriatr Soc* **62**(4) 762–769.

Livingston, G. et al. 2014. Non-pharmacological interventions for agitation in dementia: systematic review of randomised controlled trials. *Br J Psychiatry* **205**(6) 436–442.

Schneider, L. S. et al. 2006. Effectiveness of atypical antipsychotic drugs in patients with Alzheimer's disease. *New Engl J Med* **355**(15) 1525–1538.

Sink, K. M., Holden, K. F. and Yaffe, K. 2005. Pharmacological treatment of neuropsychiatric symptoms of dementia: a review of the evidence. *JAMA* **293**(5) 596–608.

Tible, O. P., Riese, F., Savaskan, E. and von Gunten, A. 2017. Best practice in the management of behavioural and psychological symptoms of dementia. *Ther Adv Neurol Disord* **10**(8) 297–309.

Van Den Wijngaart, M. A., Vernooij-Dassen, M. J. and Felling, A. J. 2007. The influence of stressors, appraisal and personal conditions on the burden of spousal caregivers of persons with dementia. *Aging Ment Health* **11**(6) 626–636.

Yaffe, K. et al. 2002. Patient and caregiver characteristics and nursing home placement in patients with dementia. *JAMA* **287**(16) 2090–2097.

Case: This 67-year-old right-handed man presented with a 2-year history of progressive memory decline. He first noticed that he required an increasing number of written reminders at work. However, his performance as an accountant was not affected. At home, his wife started writing grocery lists for him, which she had never done before. He reported difficulty coming up with words and recalling names, particularly if he had recently met the person. He was able to perform all his activities of daily living independently, except for his finances, which his children were now supervising. Under the counsel of his children, he was now considering retirement. His motor examination was unremarkable. Montreal Cognitive Assessment (MoCA) score was 24/30 due to impairments in phonemic fluency and delayed recall (he did not recall any words freely and recognized two when multiple choices were given). His brain MRI showed mild bilateral hippocampal atrophy.

After discussing the diagnosis of mild cognitive impairment and the possibility of underlying Alzheimer disease with the patient and his family, his children asked about driving. They had not noticed any changes in his driving abilities, and he had not been involved in any accidents or violations. However, given the diagnosis they wanted to prioritize his safety and preferred that he avoided driving. The patient did not agree with this, not only because he felt he could still drive but also because not driving would greatly limit his independence.

Should Safety Be Prioritized at Any Cost in This Situation?

Driving is a complex skill encompassing almost all cognitive domains, from simple attention to praxis. Deficits in any of these domains can affect the ability to drive, which can have consequences as severe as death due to accidents. However, driving remains an important factor for independence, particularly in the elderly, and taking away such privilege can affect the quality of life of patients and caregivers (Taylor and Tripodes, 2001). Therefore, while one may consider it safer to discourage driving in a patient diagnosed with mild cognitive impairment, this restriction can affect quality of life and the ability to carry on social and physical activities, which are known to be important in the management of cognitive impairment.

In this case, there were no significant risk factors to warrant the recommendation of driving cessation. A driving evaluation was recommended. This was presented as an opportunity for the patient to reassure his family he was still able to drive safely. He agreed to undergo the driving evaluation and passed it without any problems. His family was reassured about this and it was recommended to monitor him for any changes.

Discussion

Driving skills deteriorate with increasing dementia severity (Dubinsky et al., 2000). However, there is still no clear parameter to determine if a patient with cognitive impairment is safe to drive or not, so clinicians are only able to make qualitative estimates of driving risk. The elements needed to make this assessment include but are not limited to the severity of the cognitive impairment, changes in driving habits, and other factors that are not related to the neurodegenerative process but affect driving ability. Overall, clinician assessment remains the best way of predicting unsafe driving (Brown et al., 2005).

When considering the severity of cognitive impairment, the Clinical Dementia Rating (CDR) is established as useful for identifying patients at increased risk of unsafe driving. While the relative risk of failing an on-road driving test (ORDT) significantly increases with CDRs above 0, a substantial number of patients between the ranges of 0.5 (i.e., very mild) and 1 (mild) dementia will pass the ORDT. Subjects with a CDR of 0.5–1 (i.e., very mild dementia) are often considered safe for driving if no other risk factors (as described below) are reported (Iverson et al., 2010). Although performance in cognitive screening tests does not correlate with safe driving, poor performances, such a score of ≤24 on the Mini-Mental Status Exam (MMSE) or ≤12 on the MoCA, suggest unsafe driving (Esser et al., 2016). Neuropsychological evaluation yields a better assessment of executive and visuospatial abilities, which are key skills for driving. Neuropsychiatric features such as irritability, impulsivity or apathy, should also be considered when evaluating driving safety. In addition to cognitive impairment, medical conditions (e.g., hearing

Table 49.1 Caregiver questionnaire assessing driving safety

	Strongly disagree	Disagree	No opinion	Agree	Strongly agree
I have concerns about the patient's ability to drive safely.					
Others have concerns about his/her ability to drive safely.					
The patient has limited the amount of driving that he/she does.					
He/she avoids driving at night.					
He/she avoids driving in the rain.					
He/she avoids driving in busy traffic.					
The patient will drive faster than the speed limit if the patient thinks he/she won't be caught.					
The patient will run a red light if the patient thinks that he/she won't be caught.					
The patient will drive after drinking more alcohol than the patient should.					
When he/she gets angry with other drivers, the patient will honk the horn, gesture, or drive up too closely to them.					
The patient falls asleep at the wheel.					

Source: Adapted from Iverson et al. (2010).

and visual defects, motor deficits) and medications (e.g., pain medications, sleeping aids, anticholinergic burden) may affect driving safety. Assessment of sleep apnea is warranted as it can lead to impairment in arousal and attention, and impaired response selection, motor response, and decision making, which are critical for driving (Flemons et al., 1993). Complaints of excessive sleepiness or daytime fatigue should be clues to investigate for sleep apnea, but patients with dementia or chronic sleep disorders may no longer be aware of the degree of their sleep deprivation (Ohayon and Vecchierini, 2002; Strohl et al., 2013). Patients and caregivers should be specifically asked if as drivers they ever fell asleep at the wheel, or if there were near misses because of sleepiness.

The patient and the caregiver are encouraged to provide their perspectives on whether driving safety is of concern. While patient's self-rating is not accurate in determining driving safety, the caregiver's rating of marginal or unsafe is useful in identifying unsafe drivers (Iverson et al., 2010). Caregivers may hint to this by stating they no longer go with the patient in the car or they only allow the patient to drive with someone in the car. Along these lines, self-reported driving avoidance or restriction is also considered a risk factor for driving safety, even if patients do not consider their driving unsafe. Asking the patient and their caregivers to separately fill out a questionnaire surveying these changes in driving habits is a helpful assessment tool (Table 49.1). In addition, a survey of any driving incidents (e.g., traffic violations, accidents) would ideally be conducted for both the patient and their caregiver. A history of a crash or citations within the past three years is more predictive of a high risk of subsequent crashes than the presence of mild dementia alone (Iverson et al., 2010). However, it is important to take into consideration the capacity and motivations of a caregiver in providing feedback about driving. If the individual with cognitive impairment is the sole driver, caregivers may intentionally or unintentionally underreport safety concerns. Caregivers may underreport as well because of their own memory deficiencies.

Finally, formal driving evaluation, whether an ORDT or a driving simulator, is an excellent resource. The results from these evaluations support discouraging driving in those patients who are resistant to stop driving. Conversely, normal results serve to reassure concerned families the patient is still safe to drive. Independent of the method of assessment, patients who continue to drive may need to be reassessed at periods as short as six-month intervals.

Diagnosis: Mild cognitive impairment, possible Alzheimer disease

Tip: Driving abilities are important to survey at all stages of cognitive impairment. Besides the severity of cognitive impairment, changes in driving habits and traffic incidents are useful in evaluating the safety to drive. Finally, addressing manageable factors affecting driving, including sleep apnea and sedative burden from medications, is recommended.

References

Brown, L. B. et al. 2005. Prediction of on-road driving performance in patients with early Alzheimer's disease. *J Am Geriatr Soc* **53**(1) 94–98.

Dubinsky, R. M., Stein, A. C. and Lyons, K. 2000. Practice parameter: risk of driving and Alzheimer's disease (an evidence-based review): report of the quality standards subcommittee of the American Academy of Neurology. *Neurology* **54**(12) 2205–2211.

Esser, P. et al. 2016. Utility of the MOCA as a cognitive predictor for fitness to drive. *J Neurol Neurosurg Psychiatry* **87**(5) 567–568.

Flemons, W. W., Remmers, J. E. and Whitelaw, W. A. 1993. The correlation of a computer simulated driving program with polysomnographic indices and neuropsychological tests in consecutively referred patients for assessment of sleep apnea. *Sleep* **16**(8 Suppl) S71.

Iverson, D. J. et al. 2010. Practice parameter update: evaluation and management of driving risk in dementia: report of the Quality Standards Subcommittee of the American Academy of Neurology. *Neurology* **74**(16) 1316–1324.

Ohayon, M. M. and Vecchierini, M. F. 2002. Daytime sleepiness and cognitive impairment in the elderly population. *Arch Intern Med* **162**(2) 201–208.

Strohl, K. P. et al. 2013. An official American Thoracic Society Clinical Practice Guideline: sleep apnea, sleepiness, and driving risk in noncommercial drivers. An update of a 1994 Statement. *Am J Respir Crit Care Med* **187**(11) 1259–1266.

Taylor, B. D. and Tripodes, S. 2001. The effects of driving cessation on the elderly with dementia and their caregivers. *Accid Anal Prev* **33**(4) 519–528.

Case: This 77-year-old right-handed man presented to the clinic with a 15-year history of slowly progressive fatigue associated with cognitive difficulties. He reported being slow in his thinking, with difficulties concentrating and multitasking. In the past seven years, his gait slowed, balance declined, and he walked more cautiously to avoid falls. In addition, he developed urinary urgency with occasional incontinence. His neurological exam revealed bradykinesia, cogwheel rigidity and resting tremor, most prominent in the right arm. His gait was mildly wide based, slow with decreased arm swing, and he had stooped posture. On neuropsychological evaluation he was slow in his cognitive processing but, when given additional time, he performed within normal limits in all cognitive domains, including executive function. His brain MRI revealed ventriculomegaly with subcortical and periventricular white matter hyperintensities. The degree of ventriculomegaly was considered disproportionate to the degree of parenchymal atrophy (Figure 50.1). These findings led to the suspicion of normal pressure hydrocephalus (NPH).

What Do You Make of the Asymmetric Parkinsonism?

The presence of asymmetric bradykinesia, rigidity and resting tremor suggest an underlying neurodegenerative parkinsonism, most likely Parkinson disease. However, the predominance of gait over cognitive impairment in the context of a ventriculomegaly disproportionate to the extent of parenchymal atrophy raises the concern of symptomatic ventriculomegaly (i.e., hydrocephalus). More to the point, he was suspected to have NPH.

As a result, he underwent a three-day external lumbar drainage procedure with significant improvements in his gait and urinary control (Video 50.1). He reported a marked improvement in his cognitive speed, although his Mini-Mental State Examination (MMSE) score was 30/30 at his initial exam. These

benefits slowly declined in the following weeks. A decision was made to place a ventriculoperitoneal shunt. He reported benefit in his gait and cognition after the shunt, but not as prominent as he had after the lumbar drain. After six months, he felt that there was still some improvement in his gait compared to his initial assessment, but had noticed progressive decline in his gait, urinary urgency and cognitive processing speed. In addition, his tremor had worsened and was now bothersome (Video 50.2). He and his spouse were concerned about this decline and wanted to have a discussion with the neurosurgeon regarding further adjustments of the ventriculoperitoneal valve settings.

Are Further Valve Adjustments Warranted?

The initial assessment considered Parkinson disease, but hydrocephalus prevailed as the main or contributing factor to his disability. Shunting may have alleviated some symptoms associated with the hydrocephalus but would not address those secondary to the underlying neurodegeneration. While valve adjustments can be considered, additional benefits are unlikely. In addition, side effects from over drainage (e.g., orthostatic headache and subdural hematomas) may occur.

Three hundred milligrams daily of levodopa was started with moderate benefits on his tremor and gait. Subsequent adjustments of his ventriculoperitoneal valve did not provide additional benefits.

Discussion

NPH is a syndrome attributed to increased accumulation of cerebrospinal fluid in the ventricular system or subarachnoid space. The excess fluid exerts pressure on the adjacent nervous tissue, disrupting normal functioning. The clinical syndrome is described as a triad of gait impairment, urinary incontinence and cognitive impairment, associated with ventriculomegaly (Graff-

Video 50.1 The examination demonstrates the patient's gait before and after the external lumbar drain. Note the significant change in his gait speed.

Video 50.2 Evaluation done six months later shows a resting tremor, bradykinesia, and slowness in gait, with decreased arm swing.

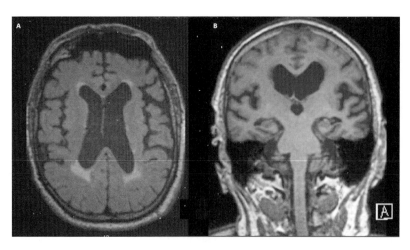

Figure 50.1 Brain MRI in this patient: (A) axial FLAIR demonstrating ventriculomegaly in addition to periventricular white matter hyperintensities; (B) coronal T1 showing ventriculomegaly, interpreted as disproportionate to the extent of cortical atrophy. Callosal angle was 88° (normal value is > 90° and, in patients with NPH, usually between 50° and 90°) (Ishii et al., 2008).

Radford and Jones, 2019). Currently, if the diversion of CSF through shunting or the removal of a large quantity of CSF improve any element of the triad, it is considered diagnostic confirmation. As such, NPH has been classically construed as a reversible form of cognitive impairment, fueling a trend for overdiagnosis and, as a result, mistreatment (Espay et al., 2017).

However, it has been established that up to two-thirds of those with initial benefit from CSF shunting show progressive deterioration by three years, despite further adjustments to the shunt settings (Espay et al., 2017). The classic literature suggests that NPH "increases the risk" for later appearance of neurodegenerative disorders. Based on the accumulated experience reported from Mayo and Cincinnati, "NPH" may more likely represent a diagnostic label that applies to hydrocephalic (NPH-like) presentations of neurodegenerative disorders (Klassen and Ahlskog, 2011; Starr et al., 2014). While hydrocephalus can be a contributing factor to the clinical neurodegenerative disorder, it is most likely a consequence of it and therefore holds no direct etiologic relevance. Therefore, shunting may provide only temporary relief; in some instances, it may hasten the clinical deterioration. Thus, the diagnostic suspicion of NPH should be approached with caution, as ventriculomegaly and the classic triad of NPH (i.e., cognitive impairment, loss of urinary control and gait impairment) are not specific (Oliveira et al., 2019). Uncovering atypical clinical features on exam, such as hallucinations, REM sleep behavior disorder or oculomotor abnormalities, can help to establish an underlying neurodegenerative disorder. In addition, other factors associated with impaired CSF reabsorption may cause hydrocephalus, including

prior subarachnoid hemorrhage or meningitis, and impaired glymphatic flow (Ringstad et al., 2017). Untreated sleep obstructive apnea has also been suggested as a contributing factor of hydrocephalus, affecting flow through increased raising jugular venous and intracranial pressure (Roman et al., 2018). Therefore, it is important to evaluate for sleep apnea in this group of patients.

When discussing the option of ventriculoperitoneal shunting, the possibility of suboptimal or transient rather than sustained benefit (given the high likelihood of an underlying neurodegeneration, most often dementia with Lewy bodies, Alzheimer disease or progressive supranuclear palsy) may need to be discussed (Starr et al., 2014). Response beyond three years is limited to a third of those undergoing the procedure after qualifying for it on the basis of adequate response to large volume tap or external lumbar drainage (Espay et al., 2017). Subjective and objective assessment of symptoms are recommended before and after either of these testing procedures. A significant benefit after this procedure increases the likelihood for at least short-term response to ventriculoperitoneal shunt (Halperin et al., 2015).

Diagnosis: Parkinson disease presenting with hydrocephalus, suspected to represent NPH

Tip: NPH is often a presentation of neurodegenerative disorders – even if suspected on inspection "disproportionate" to the extent of parenchymal atrophy. While shunting may provide symptomatic benefit, most likely to gait, the benefits may not be sustained. It is also important to suspect sleep apnea.

References

Espay, A. J. et al. 2017. Deconstructing normal pressure hydrocephalus: ventriculomegaly as early sign of neurodegeneration. *Ann Neurol* **82**(4) 503–513.

Graff-Radford, N. R. and Jones, D. T. 2019. Normal pressure hydrocephalus. *Continuum* **25**(1) 165–186.

Halperin, J. J. et al. 2015. Practice guideline: idiopathic normal pressure hydrocephalus: response to shunting and predictors of response: report of the Guideline Development, Dissemination, and Implementation Subcommittee of the American Academy of Neurology. *Neurology* **85**(23) 2063–2071.

Ishii, K. et al. 2008. Clinical impact of the callosal angle in the diagnosis of idiopathic normal pressure hydrocephalus. *Eur Radiol* **18**(11) 2678–2683.

Klassen, B. T. and Ahlskog, J. E. 2011. Normal pressure hydrocephalus: how often does the diagnosis hold water? *Neurology* **77**(12) 1119–1125.

Oliveira, L. M., Nitrini, R. and Roman, G. C. 2019. Normal-pressure hydrocephalus: a critical review. *Dement Neuropsychol* **13**(2) 133–143.

Ringstad, G., Vatnehol, S. A. S. and Eide, P. K. 2017. Glymphatic MRI in idiopathic normal pressure hydrocephalus. *Brain* **140**(10) 2691–2705.

Roman, G. C., Verma, A. K., Zhang, Y. J. and Fung, S. H. 2018. Idiopathic normal-pressure hydrocephalus and obstructive sleep apnea are frequently associated: a prospective cohort study. *J Neurol Sci* **395** 164–168.

Starr, B. W., Hagen, M. C. and Espay, A. J. 2014. Hydrocephalic Parkinsonism: lessons from normal pressure hydrocephalus mimics. *J Clin Mov Disord* **1** 2.

Case: This 70-year-old right-handed man presented with a 4-year history of worsening forgetfulness. Since his retirement as a lawyer he noticed increasing difficulties recalling recent conversations and finding words. His family reported he was unintentionally repeating questions and stories. In addition, he was not as active as before and spent more time watching TV. One year earlier, he discussed his concerns with his primary care physician whose evaluation revealed a Mini-Mental State Examination score (MMSE) of 24/30, unremarkable screening labs, and a brain MRI which showed mild generalized atrophy. He was told he had mild cognitive impairment (MCI) which is considered a predementia stage. He was on donepezil 10 mg daily and memantine 10 mg twice daily, with no meaningful changes in his cognition or function.

On exam, he was alert and oriented. His speech was fluent with occasional pauses between words. The remainder of his exam was unremarkable, except for mild difficulties with hearing. The Montreal Cognitive Assessment (MoCA) score was 23/30 due to impairments in trail making, sentence repetition, and delayed recall (he did not recall any words freely and recognized only one when multiple choices were given). His brain MRI revealed generalized atrophy, including both hippocampi, as well as mild subcortical white matter hyperintensities (Figure 51.1).

When discussing the assessment of MCI, the patient and his family interpreted it as confirmation of what they have been previously told: MCI is a preliminary stage of dementia, which they equated to Alzheimer disease (AD), an incurable disease.

How Do You Address the Patient's Concerns?

The first step in the discussion is to clarify that the characterization of cognitive impairment includes two separate designations: one indicating degree (severity) of cognitive impairment and a second that identifies etiologies, which are often multiple. Terms that indicate severity are often based on the Clinical Dementia Rating scale (CDR) which incorporate three neuropsychological ratings (memory, orientation, and judgment) and three functional ratings (activities in the community, activities at home, and self-care) derived from formal testing and clinical interviews (Hughes et al., 1982). Each of the six domains are rated independently and also integrated into a weighted calculation that computes an overall designation (www.alz.washington.edu/cdrnacc.html) (Table 51.1). It is important to recognize that there may be a very significant neuropsychological impairment, for example an amnestic syndrome, but depending on its impact on function, a person may still be rated as having mild cognitive impairment. The CDR is generally applicable to the all neurodegenerative disorders, but there are modifications for primary progressive aphasias and frontotemporal dementia to account for the impact of language and behavior in these conditions. The terms used to identify cognitive impairment reflect the current view of neurodegenerative disorders as chronic diseases, in which pathology accrues over decades and may not initially manifest with cognitive symptoms or functional impact. Additionally, for patients and families it is important to clarify that mild dementia still indicates severe cognitive impairment. The term "mild" is a qualifier of dementia. Dementia implies a significant functional impact, first on activities in the community, followed by function at home, and finally on self-care. Mild cognitive impairment is the term that captures less severe cognitive impairment and less significant impact on function.

The determination of the causes of cognitive impairment at any stage involves consideration of both nonneurodegenerative and neurodegenerative conditions. In addition, multiple neurodegenerative pathologies may coexist. In general, progressive decline over time is associated with neurodegenerative pathology. In addition, aging itself is not associated with significant cognitive decline (see Case 1). However, neither a designation of MCI nor dementia necessarily implies a progressive disorder. While older adults with MCI are three times more likely to progress to dementia in the next two to five years, between 15 and 50 percent of patients remain stable or improve, even revert to normal, if treatable factors are identified and addressed or even spontaneously (Petersen et al., 2018). Moreover, in this case, underlying AD has not been established by either CSF biomarkers or amyloid imaging.

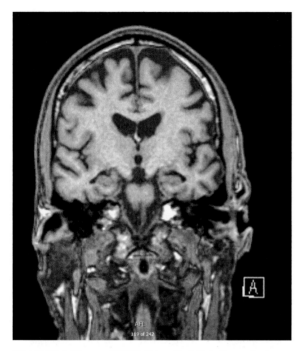

Figure 51.1 T1 coronal MRI in this patient. Note the cortical atrophy, including involvement of both hippocampi.

Further questioning revealed he snored and had been diagnosed with mild obstructive sleep apnea five years ago. However, the mask (i.e., CPAP machine) was uncomfortable, and he did not want to use it. In addition, he noted some difficulties in his hearing which he attributed to aging and which had never been addressed. Cerebrospinal fluid AD biomarkers showed elevation of p-tau (73.02 pg/ml) and a decrease in amyloid β-42/total tau index (ATI) (0.7), which were consistent with AD

Now That You Have Established He Has Alzheimer Disease, Is There Anything Else Left to Do?

Although the diagnosis of AD can account for his cognitive impairment, other factors, including his sleep apnea and hearing impairment, could be contributing to some of his symptoms and therefore need to be addressed. In addition, his routine and sedentary lifestyle were not beneficial for his brain health. Therefore, he should be encouraged to exercise and engage in social activities, as well as picking up a new hobby that can challenge him cognitively. The impact of these lifestyle changes is often underappreciated by the patients and their families, and the relevance they may have toward improving symptoms and potentially ameliorating progression of the disease needs to be emphasized.

As a side note, the patient should be made aware that there is no clear evidence supporting the use of donepezil or memantine in improving MCI or reducing the rate of progression to dementia.

Discussion

The current lack of disease-modifying medications specific for AD create the false impression that nothing can be done to treat this disorder. This leads to delays in the pursuit of diagnosis from patients and anchoring bias among physicians, representing a missed opportunity to improve cognition and enact dietary and lifestyle choices that may decrease the rate of decline. Understanding that management of cognitive impairment goes beyond the use of cholinesterase inhibitors and memantine is one of the most important factors in caring for these patients.

The approach to the modification of cognitive decline focuses on three factors that affect cognition: reducing brain damage, addressing behavioral symptoms, and increasing cognitive reserve (Table 51.2). Patients with a recent diagnosis of cognitive impairment and their families may be the keen to explore these opportunities if the message that it is never too late to start is emphasized. In addition, this approach is also recommended in subjects without cognitive impairment who want to decrease the risk of developing cognitive impairment.

The recommended practice is to evaluate potentially treatable factors associated with cognitive impairment, as well as establishing a neurodegenerative disease(s) as the underlying etiology. Periodic screening and monitoring of these variables is strongly recommended given their independent role in cognition. Behavioral symptoms (e.g., depression, anxiety) are common in MCI and may be associated with greater functional impairment and increased risk of progression from MCI to dementia (Petersen et al., 2018). Both nonpharmacological and pharmacological strategies may be warranted.

In addition to addressing factors that are detrimental to the brain, strategies to improve brain health or cognitive reserve should be emphasized. These include several lifestyle interventions, such as aerobic exercise, socialization, and engaging in a wide variety of novel activities, all of which are related to

Table 51.1 Clinical Dementia Rating Scale

Impairment	None	Questionable	Mild	Moderate	Severe
CDR score	0	0.5	1	2	3
Memory	No memory loss or slight inconstant forgetfulness	Consistent slight forgetfulness; partial recollection of events	Moderate memory loss; more marked for recent events; defect interferes with everyday activities	Severe memory loss; only highly learned material retained; new material rapidly lost	Severe memory loss; only fragments remain
Orientation	Fully oriented	Fully oriented or slight difficulty with time relationships	Moderate difficulty with time relationships; oriented for place at examination; may have geographic disorientation elsewhere	Severe difficulty with time relationships; usually disoriented in time, often to place	Oriented to person only
Judgment and problem solving	Solves everyday problems and handles business and financial affairs well; judgment good in relation to past performance	Slight impairment to solving problems, similarities, differences	Moderate difficulty in handling problems, similarities, differences; social judgment usually maintained	Severely impaired in handling problems, similarities, differences; social judgment usually impaired	Unable to make judgments or solve problems
Community affairs	Independent function at usual level in job, shopping, volunteer and social groups	Slight impairment in these activities	Unable to function independently at these activities though may still be engaged in some; appears normal to casual inspection	No pretense of independent function outside of home; appears well enough to be taken to functions outside of family home	No pretense of independent function outside of home; appears too ill to be taken to functions outside a family home
Home and hobbies	Life at home, hobbies, intellectual interests well maintained	Life at home, hobbies, intellectual interests slightly impaired	Mild but definite impairment of function at home; more difficult chores abandoned; more complicated hobbies and interests abandoned	Only simple chores preserved; very restricted interests, poorly maintained	No significant function in home
Personal care	Fully capable of self-care	Fully capable of self-care	Needs prompting	Requires assistance in dressing, hygiene, keeping of personal effects	Requires much help with personal care; frequent incontinence

Table 51.2 Suggested strategies aiming to improve cognitive decline

Category	Strategies
Reducing brain damage	• Avoid medications with sedative or anticholinergic side effects • Avoid smoking • Reduce alcohol intake to ≤ 2 drinks/week (1 drink = 6 oz wine, 12 oz beer, 1 shot of liquor) • Suspect and treat sleep apnea • Employ good sleep hygiene • Reduce blood sugar and optimize treatment of diabetes • Optimize vascular risk factors (e.g., hypertension, hypercholesterolemia) • Screen for and correct (orthostatic) hypotension • Treat associated metabolic, endocrine and vitamin abnormalities • Maintain BMI < 25
Address behavioral symptoms	• Treat mood disorders with SSRI/SNRI associated with the least anticholinergic and sedative side effects • Avoid benzodiazepines for treatment of anxiety
Improve cognitive reserve	• Screen for and address hearing loss • Urge aerobic exercise, optimally 5–7 days/week • Encourage socialization • Establish new hobbies and pursuits emphasizing activities that are intrinsically of interest and instill a sense of awe or inspiration • Recommend the MIND dietary guidelines

evolutionary-conserved triggers for expansion of dendritic connections and possibly neurogenesis (Fotuhi et al., 2012; Karssemeijer et al., 2017). Although exact dosing and intensity of aerobic exercise is not yet clear, aerobic activity at least twice a week has demonstrated cognitive benefit among MCI patients (Petersen et al., 2018). Combined cognitive and aerobic activity may be more robust in enhancing overall cognition, activities of daily living (ADLs), and mood. It has also been suggested that exercise increases brain volume, including in the hippocampus, although confirmatory evidence is awaited (Fotuhi et al., 2012).

In addition to cognition, exercise also improves cardiovascular function and mood, which may have additional positive effects on cognition (Livingston et al., 2017). Cognitive decline is often associated with withdrawal from social activities and hobbies, frequently resulting in a routine deprived of activities. Social isolation might also result in cognitive inactivity, which is linked to faster cognitive decline and low mood (Kuiper et al., 2015). Improving cognitive stimulation, particularly through social activities and stimulating new hobbies, has also been shown to reduce decline and improve cognition (Akbaraly et al., 2009). Novel and engaging activities should be prioritized over "brain games," computer-based drills, or crossword puzzles, These can be as simple as listening to new music, walking on a new route, engaging in creative arts, or learning new things related to prior

interests. It is bet to start with a small, weekly commitment that can be slowly increased.

Dietary changes are often encouraged, particularly if they relate to the management of a concomitant condition. However, while multiple diets have shown to decrease the risk of developing cognitive impairment, the extent to which they delay cognitive decline remains to be determined. However, similar to exercise, given their benefit on overall health, the MIND diet has been favored (Morris et al., 2015a, 2015b). Unless a deficiency is identified, there is no sufficient evidence supporting dietary supplements such as fish oil or vitamins (Livingston et al., 2017).

Diagnosis: Mild cognitive impairment with biomarker-positive Alzheimer disease pathology; sleep apnea, hearing loss, and sedentary lifestyle may also be contributors

Tip: The management of cognitive impairment goes beyond the diagnosis of a neurodegenerative process and prescription of cholinesterase inhibitors or memantine. The promotion of bran health and cognitive reserve are fundamental in the care of patients with cognitive impairment.

References

Akbaraly, T. N. et al. 2009. Leisure activities and the risk of dementia in the elderly: results from the Three-City Study. *Neurology* **73**(11) 854–861.

Fotuhi, M., Do, D. and Jack, C. 2012. Modifiable factors that alter the size of the hippocampus with ageing. *Nature Reviews Neurology* **8** 189.

Hughes, C. P. et al. 1982. A new clinical scale for the staging of dementia. *Br J Psychiatry* **140** 566–572.

Karssemeijer, E. G. A. et al. 2017. Positive effects of combined cognitive and physical exercise training on cognitive function in older adults with mild cognitive impairment or dementia: a meta-analysis. *Ageing Res Rev* **40** 75–83.

Kuiper, J. S. et al. 2015. Social relationships and risk of dementia: a systematic review and meta-analysis of longitudinal cohort studies. *Ageing Res Rev* **22** 39–57.

Livingston, G. et al. 2017. Dementia prevention, intervention, and care. *Lancet* **390**(10113) 2673–2734.

Morris, M. C. et al. 2015a. MIND diet slows cognitive decline with aging. *Alzheimers Dement* **11**(9) 1015–1022.

Morris, M. C. et al. 2015b. MIND diet associated with reduced incidence of Alzheimer's disease. *Alzheimers Dement* **11**(9) 1007–1014.

Petersen, R. C. et al. 2018. Practice guideline update summary: mild cognitive impairment: report of the Guideline Development, Dissemination, and Implementation Subcommittee of the American Academy of Neurology. *Neurology* **90**(3) 126–135.

Index